NATURAL REMEDIE!
Mental an
Emotional Health

T0272463

"For all things herbal and healing, I am an avid Brigitte Mars fan. In this work with Chrystle Fiedler, Brigitte weaves into herbal healing magic, spirit, clinical science, practical applications, and guidance like few others. Brigitte's work is about transformation, inspiration, and guiding people in how to become their best self, based on real world clinical experience. Brigitte and Chrystle's guidance to improve mental and emotional health is so needed in our current times. This work will be an invaluable tool for those willing to start that journey toward true well-being."

ROY UPTON, PRESIDENT OF THE
AMERICAN HERBAL PHARMACOPOEIA

"For those interested in holistic self-care, this is the one reference book they should have in their home library. It is comprehensive, practical, and user-friendly."

ROBERT S. IVKER, D.O., COFOUNDER OF THE AMERICAN
BOARD OF INTEGRATIVE HOLISTIC MEDICINE
AND AUTHOR OF *SINUS SURVIVAL*

"An excellent and straightforward book for the lay person looking to support their nervous system for a long and healthy life. The authors have covered a full spectrum of natural therapies to do just that. A must-have book on anyone's shelf."

FEATHER JONES, RH(AHG), AUTHOR OF
THE MEDICINAL HERB HANDBOOK

"We often forget that the mind and emotions need just as much care and healing as the physical body. This entire book is a panacea for challenging times."

EMMA FARRELL, AUTHOR OF *JOURNEYS WITH PLANT SPIRITS*

NATURAL REMEDIES FOR
Mental and Emotional Health

Holistic Methods and Techniques
for a Happy and Healthy Mind

BRIGITTE MARS, A.H.G.
and
CHRYSTLE FIEDLER

Healing Arts Press
Rochester, Vermont

Healing Arts Press
One Park Street
Rochester, Vermont 05767
www.HealingArtsPress.com

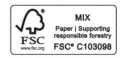

Healing Arts Press is a division of Inner Traditions International

Originally published in 2015 by Fair Winds Press, an imprint of The Quarto Group, under the title *The Home Reference to Holistic Health and Healing*.

Note to the reader: *This book is intended to be an informational guide. The remedies, approaches, and techniques described herein are meant to supplement, and not to be a substitute for, professional medical care or treatment. They should not be used to treat a serious ailment without prior consultation with a qualified health care professional.*

Cataloging-in-Publication Data for this title is available from the Library of Congress

ISBN 978-1-64411-786-6 (print)
ISBN 978-1-64411-787-3 (ebook)

Printed and bound in the United States by Lake Book Manufacturing, LLC

10 9 8 7 6 5 4 3 2 1

Text design and layout by Priscilla Harris Baker
This book was typeset in Garamond Premier Pro, with Futura and URW DIN used as display typefaces.

To send correspondence to the author of this book, mail a first-class letter to the author c/o Inner Traditions • Bear & Company, One Park Street, Rochester, VT 05767, and we will forward the communication, or contact the author directly at **brigittemars.com** and **chrystlefiedlerbooks.com**.

From Brigitte:
This book is dedicated to my daughters, Sunflower
Sparkle Mars and Rainbeau Harmony Mars; to
three amazing grandchildren, Jade Destiny Mars,
Solwyn Forest Stegall, and Luna Zara Mars;
to my son-in-law, Mitch Stegall, and to
Nisa Mars Counter and, of course,
the om-azing BethyLoveLight.
For the highest good!

From Chrystle:
For Glynis Sherwood and Aubrey Cannata,
who helped me navigate the road less traveled.
It has made all the difference.

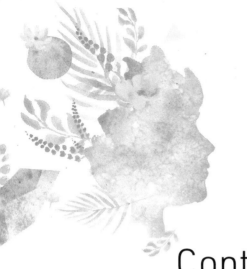

Contents

🌿

PART 1

REBALANCING
Supporting Mental Health
and the Brain

PART 4

REVITALIZATION

Boosting Mental and Emotional Health

PART 5

REMEDIES

Therapies and Herbs to Support Mental and Emotional Health

Foreword

Rosemary Gladstar

I am always moved by the grace, wisdom, joie de vivre, and charismatic charm that Brigitte Mars brings to life and shares so generously with others through her teachings, books, and classes. The numerous books she's written on herbs and natural health are among my favorite herbal references and are frequently listed on my recommended reading lists for students. They are also on the rather hefty shelf of go-to books I refer to most often when seeking reliable herbal information. Brigitte not only writes from her years of experience as an herbal practitioner but also weaves together a wide spectrum of natural healing modalities she's integrated into her practice. Her books are always comprehensive, well-researched, user-friendly, and practical.

Chrystle Fiedler, too, has had a lifelong love affair with herbs and natural remedies and has combined her interest in alternative medicine with her excellent communication and writing skills. She's authored several excellent books on natural healing, including *Beat Sugar Addiction Now!* and *The Complete Idiot's Guide to Natural Remedies,* dozens of articles on natural health for national and international publications, and a natural remedies mystery series for Gallery and Pocket Books. Together, this dyamic team coauthored two excellent resources, *The*

Country Almanac of Home Remedies and *Natural Remedies for Mental and Emotional Health.*

Natural Remedies for Mental and Emotional Health is quite simply one of the most comprehensive self-care books on the subject of mental and emotional well-being. It contains a wealth of important information, tools, and insightful suggestions to help one deal with the daily stresses of modern life as well the illnesses and imbalances that arise from an overly stressed nervous system. The subject matter is extensive, covering the whole gamut of mental, emotional, and nervous system disorders and each topic is covered with a wealth of information including herbal, homeopathic, and flower essences; supplements; and lifestyle suggestions.

Not only useful and practical, *Natural Remedies for Mental and Emotional Health* is also uplifting to read, in part because it brings hope to a rather dense subject and also because both Brigitte and Chrystle bring such a wealth of experience and skills to the subject and share them generously and joyfully with others. They lighten the very subjects of depression, mental stress, and emotional imbalance with their deep insights, compassion, and wisdom.

It is estimated that more than 100 million Americans suffer from stress-related problems and that stress-related issues account for more than 80 percent of doctor's visits. Yet many of these issues and visits can be circumvented by understanding the underlying problem(s) and are often resolved by natural remedies and lifestyle changes. Although there are undoubtedly times when medical intervention is necessary and lifesaving—and this book clearly points to that direction when needed—most of the daily stress-related issues we encounter are safely and effectively treated by less invasive and equally effective home remedies.

Mental and emotional well-being is as essential and as important as physical health for living a harmonious and productive life, yet emotional/mental health is often overlooked or trivialized. Our go-go culture doesn't allow a lot of time for nurturing the soul, or taking time out to care for one's spirit. The healing power of herbs and other natural practices can help do just that. Natural cures help soothe stress, ease anxiety, and boost mood, immunity, mental acuity, and energy, and they make room in our lives for greater joy and happiness. This book is filled with the best suggestions for just how to do that, and equally important, it gives practical, easy to follow, step-by-step instructions.

Although Americans are just waking up to the power of herbal and natural medicine, these practices are as old as civilization itself. According to the World Health Organization, 80 percent of the world uses herbal and natural remedies as a primary source of health care. *The Natural Pharmacy,* a popular book written by several experts on natural healing, reports that one out of every three adult Americans uses complementary and alternative medical care.

Holistic healing works in myriad ways to support mental health and emotional well-being, which, in turn, support our physical health as well. For example, learning how to naturally manage stress, the root of most modern illnesses, will help you not only feel better today but may also help prevent it from manifesting into another illness, such as heart disease or stroke, down the line.

Herbal and natural cures create a foundation of wellness by addressing the root of chronic health problems, which can include lifestyle choices, environmental factors, allergies, heavy metal toxicity, neurotransmitter deficiency, trauma, and yeast overgrowth. If genetics play a part in our conditions, we need to work in closer relationship with nature to overcome that adversity. *Natural Remedies for Mental and Emotional Health* is resplendent with lifestyle and practical suggestions that can begin the healing process if you are willing.

There is no denying that conventional (allopathic) medicine is making amazing progress in the twenty-first century and is an essential path of treatment if you have severe mental and emotional challenges. While this book makes clear that any life-threatening illness needs to be treated by a competent health professional, it also makes clear that herbs, natural remedies, whole foods, and lifestyle modifications are the medicine of the home, helping us to be more self-reliant and proactive in our own health care. Problems such as stress, anxiety, mild depression, low energy and immunity, and sleep and memory issues are among the many imbalances that can be effectively, safely, and inexpensively treated at home. *Natural Remedies for Mental and Emotional Health* shows us exactly how and when to do this, and does so with great compassion and care.

Brigitte and Chrystle are long-time soul sisters when it comes to herbal and holistic medicine. So, I have no doubt that you'll benefit from their wise, health-giving, joy-full advice. Like each of their other books, *Natural Remedies for Mental and Emotional Health* is written in that eminently practical and self-empowering manner that's a signature of their work. Read, practice, enjoy, and be at peace.

In joy,
Rosemary Gladstar

Rosemary Gladstar is internationally renowned in the field of modern herbalism for her technical knowledge and stewardship in the global herbalist community. She has been learning, teaching, and writing about herbs for more than forty years and is the author of eleven books. Her works include *Medicinal Herbs: A Beginners Guide, Herbal Healing for Women, Rosemary Gladstar's Herbal Recipes for Vibrant Health,* and *The Science and Art of Herbalism.* She also created an in-depth home study course and is a founder and president of United Plant Savers and founder and past director of the International Herb Symposium.

A Holistic Approach to Mental and Emotional Well-Being

G reetings! Get ready to learn hundreds of natural remedies that support the betterment of your brain, nervous system, and emotional body as well as the greening of our planet so that you can be your brightest self for the highest good.

So many people today suffer from stress, depression, anxiety, and other psychological and emotional issues that can drain the joy from life. We grow through the hardships in life, but they can be incapacitating when we have a job to do, children to raise, bills to pay, and all the rigors of life before us. Though medications are one way to manage our mental health, they can take their toll, leading to physical side effects such as low energy, diminished libido, weight gain, organ damage, addiction, and decreased immunity. The good news is that we exist in a time when we can combine myriad modalities to help heal ourselves and the planet!

Natural Remedies for Mental and Emotional Health offers time-tested, natural methods to help you manage mental and emotional challenges as well as certain neurological disorders. Here, through the lens of science, history, heritage, and nature, we will explore a full range of simple natural remedies—lifestyle choices, nutrition, medicinal herbs, essential oils, vitamins and other supplements, homeopathy, flower essences, color therapy, and more—that you can use to nourish and support your body and mind so that each challenge becomes an opportunity to be stronger than ever.

A Brief History of Natural Cures for Mental and Emotional Health

Methods for treating mental disorders have varied through the ages. Asclepius (who practiced around 130 BCE and is considered one of the fathers of medicine) restored mental and physical balance with massage, fresh air, diet, exercise, and dream interpretation. He was one of the first to release insane people from the confinements of dark cellars and recommended calming herbs, soothing music, and exercise to improve attention and memory.

Hippocrates placed the site of mental functioning in the brain and speculated that those with mental illness were imbalanced in the humors: bile, wind, and phlegm. He introduced the terms *melancholy* and *mania*.

During the Middle Ages, many traditions ascribed supernatural causes to mental diseases, including evil spirits, the stars, and wicked spells. During the Renaissance, the emphasis shifted toward more natural causes of mental illness, though there was little change in the actual treatment.

Throughout history, depression and other mental illnesses have often been treated with abuse: whipping, bloodletting, exorcism, cold water treatments, isolation, and more. Thankfully, kindness has mostly replaced brutality.

Today, we know that mental, emotional, and neurological disorders arise from a multiplicity of factors, from developmental differences to neurotransmitter and hormone imbalances to trauma, inflammation, blood sugar dysregulation, food allergies, yeast overgrowth, heavy metal and/or chemical toxin exposure, nutritional deficiencies, and more. We also know that physical conditions can contribute to mental and emotional imbalances, and mental and emotional imbalances, in turn, can affect the physical body.

Numerous rigorous clinical studies have proved the efficacy of natural cures for improving mental and emotional health, adding to the already burgeoning wealth of knowledge we have about natural medicines, first as folk remedies, now as mainstream medicine. In 1978, West Germany appointed a panel of experts, called Commission E, to study herbs for different health conditions, a key step in our modern scientific understanding of natural remedies. In 1999, the National Center for Complementary and Integrative Health (NCCIH) was founded and awarded its first research grant. Since then, scientific attention to holistic care has only grown.

We have also learned that many of our neurotransmitters are made in the gut. Therefore, diet and digestive health can play a crucial role in emotional and mental well-being. This knowledge has led us to the understanding that consuming foods that we are allergic or sensitive to, digestive disorders, overuse of antibiotics, yeast overgrowth (also called candidiasis), and inflammation affect not only the physical body but the mind and emotions as well. Common food allergens—gluten, dairy, corn, soy, shellfish, yeast—can trigger inflammation in the gut, which can trigger an autoimmune response, mental/emotional disharmony, and brain inflammation. Eating a lot of processed foods and sugar or overusing antibiotics will destroy healthy microflora and breed bad bacteria and yeast. We've also learned that the foods we are allergic to are often the foods we crave. Getting off allergens and avoiding overuse of yeast producing foods can make a world of difference to our mental and emotional health.

The Value of Holistic Care

Though life on this planet can be fraught with perils that affect not only our physical but mental, emotional, and neurological well-being, there are many remedies that have been used by millions of people for thousands of years that can contribute to our overall health, as well as a healthier planet. More people than ever before are turning to natural remedies. According to NCCIH, more than 42 percent of Americans use integrative medicine, which combines alternative and conventional medicine.

It's no surprise. Natural remedies work *with* the body's own innate processes to speed healing and build resilience instead of suppressing symptoms with medications. This is why most natural remedies are safe when used as directed (which is why it's often important to seek professional guidance). Herbs and supplements are also far less likely to cause problems with addiction and often have less side effects than medications. Many natural remedies are produced by ethical companies that support environmental and humanitarian practices such as recycling, using renewable resources, and supporting indigenous communities. These companies recognize that the health of our planet is intrinsically tied to our own health.

While this book is not meant to replace competent medical care, it shares the wisdom of numerous natural remedies and lifestyle techniques that can help lift our spirits, calm anxiety, improve mood, overcome grief, increase sleep, enhance intelligence, and even improve neurological conditions. What goes on in your mind is certainly affected by the state of your body and taking care of one will help the other.

Specialists often filter your ailments through their expertise. Say you have a headache. A chiropractor might believe it's due to a pinched nerve, while an ear nose and throat doctor may think you have a sinus infection or an eye doctor may assume your headaches are caused by eye strain. In truth, you may be stressed, anxious, and out of balance and need to incorporate wellness practices like meditation, mindfulness, and breathwork into your life along with dietary and lifestyle changes to find relief and healing. This is why a holistic approach to health and well-being can be invaluable and why holistic physicians and health care providers—who look at the whole you rather than you as the sum of your parts—are essential allies.

It's all connected—body, mind, spirit, humanity, and the world we live in. We often ignore our mind-body connection, forget to nurture and nourish ourselves, and become out of balance. We invite you to join us on this journey to explore how you can achieve a happier, healthier lifestyle. It's a virtuous circle of positivity, healing, and well-being.

How to Use This Book

Think of *Natural Remedies for Mental and Emotional Health* as your new mind-body-spirit companion on the path, offering specific advice and information that you can use right now to feel better and enjoy life more. Each chapter begins with an overview of a particular condition affecting mental or emotional health. Next, you'll learn about the types of natural remedies and therapies that can help relieve symptoms and restore balance.

Boxes throughout alert you to information you need to know, illuminate the text, and guide you on your journey to health and well-being:

🔖 **Mother Nature's News:** Timely studies that show the effectiveness of natural cures.

👎 **Skip This!** Practices to avoid.

💡 **Good to Know!** Simple remedies, surprising information, and important facts.

❗ **Cure Caution:** Warnings to note and how to know when you need professional help.

You will also find a treasure trove of information about herbs, supplements, homeopathy, and essential oils in part 5.

As a general rule, taking a holistic approach by using appropriate natural remedies, eating a diet high in plant-based organic foods, and becoming more active is the best prescription for improved health and immunity.

To find the remedies and therapies that work best for you, we suggest keeping a planner or journal in which you can list the specific interventions you'd like to try. We also suggest using a yellow highlighter to note things in the book you want to remember and perhaps look into more deeply (yellow is a good color for improving memory). Then, as you begin to put your protocol into action, take notes on how it's working. Keeping a designated journal to record your progress can be extremely helpful in your journey to self-healing.

But before you get started, please read the section below on safety and refer to it as needed.

Safety First

Before beginning any program of natural remedies, please heed a few cautions:

► Make sure your health care professional is aware of any remedies you are using, including herbs, vitamins, and other drugs.

► If you're on medication, stay on it unless otherwise instructed by your doctor.

► If you're on medication, talk to your health care practitioner about any possible contraindications before making any dietary changes or beginning to take any remedies or supplements. Mixing natural remedies with prescription drugs can cause exacerbated or unpredictable effects.

► Likewise, if you are pregnant or nursing, talk to your health care practitioner about any possible contraindications before making any dietary changes or beginning to take any remedies or supplements.

- If you are taking pharmaceuticals and herbs concurrently, separate your intake of each by at least three hours.
- When you first start using a new remedy, it may be wise to build up to the full recommended dose over a period of time rather than making an abrupt introduction.
- If you're taking medication for a particular ailment, you shouldn't also take herbs for that same ailment without first checking with your health care practitioner, or you might be giving yourself a double dose.
- If you are reducing pharmaceuticals, consider taking a vitamin C and B-complex supplement, which can aid in detoxification.
- No amount of medicine, whether it be pharmaceutical or naturopathic, can fully rectify the harm caused by poor diet, lack of sleep, and lack of physical activity. Take care of your body.

Make Changes Slowly

As you make your way through the suggestions in this book, choose the strategies that suit you and adjust as needed. Listen to your own wisdom about your body. Tune in to your cycles. Instead of rushing through your day and life, slow down and allow yourself to find your true rhythm.

Enjoy this guided journey to a healthy mind, psyche, and emotional being, all of which are affected by the healthy (or unhealthy) ways we treat our body. Learn how to use simple, time-tested techniques to feel and heal. Thank you for this opportunity to be guides on the path of well-being.

Peace and blessings on your journey!

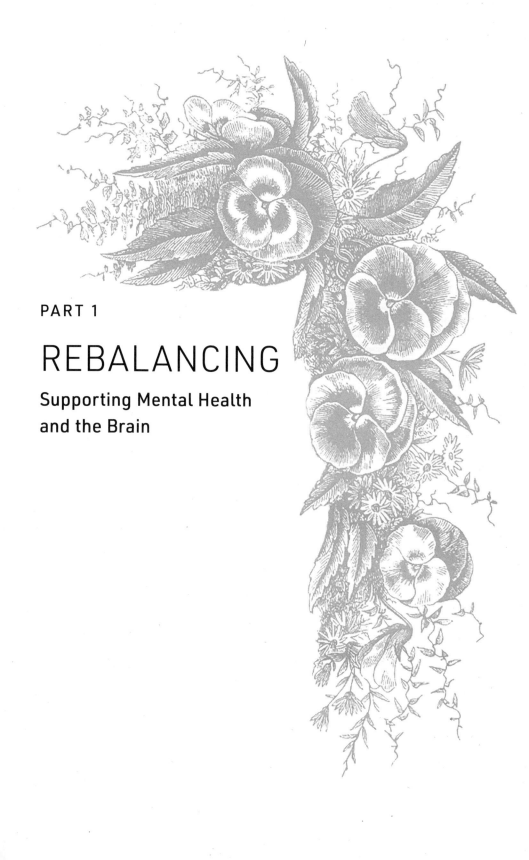

PART 1

REBALANCING

**Supporting Mental Health
and the Brain**

1
Stress

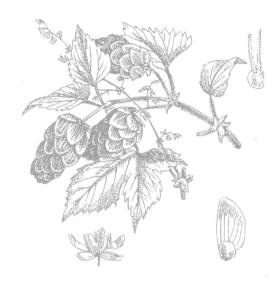

One word frees us of all the weight and pain in life: That word is love.

SOPHOCLES

Learning how to manage stress and stressful situations is one of the most important tasks on our journey to a happier life. Stress is caused by anything that disturbs our serenity and makes us feel unsafe. From the economy, technology, politics, and the state of the world to relationships, childcare, money, living situations, or illness, large and small changes alike (even positive ones) cause stress. Most of us think of stress as a necessary nuisance, but we rarely examine the cost it has on our lives, our health, and the way it causes "dis-ease" in the body.

It's easy when we're stressed to stop doing good things for ourselves. Instead, think of it as an opportunity to take better care of yourself and focus on self-care. Though stress may be unavoidable, we can come through most ordeals if they are balanced by good nutrition, exercise, useful natural remedies and therapies, rest, and spiritual or mindfulness practice. And consider taking a break from the news and social media for a while!

The Body's Response to Stress

Feeling stressed out activates the fight-or-flight response, which means hormones such as adrenaline and cortisol are released in the body. When this happens, heart rate increases so that blood is available to supply the muscles, respiratory rate and sweat production accelerate, and blood sugar levels elevate as the liver releases stored glucose into the bloodstream.

Ideally, we would experience stress and relax once the danger was over. But because we have a central cortex, stressful memories and thoughts and the feelings they provoke have a long shelf life, leaving us chronically stressed, impairing immune system function, and causing inflammation in the body, which can lead to chronic diseases like heart disease, hypertension, and diabetes. Chronic muscle tension makes us more armored because we hold our muscles tightly, which can decrease circulation and impair digestion.

Over time, chronic stress can affect mood and cognitive function and contribute to erratic behavior and even more emotional upheaval.

Signs That a Person Might Be in Emotional Trouble

- ▶ Undereating or overeating
- ▶ Sleeping too much or not enough
- ▶ Paranoia
- ▶ Thoughts of death or suicide that persist
- ▶ Lowered or excessive sex drive
- ▶ Excessive fatigue or hyperactivity
- ▶ Feeling of hopelessness
- ▶ Inability to control emotions; prone to tears or temper at slight provocation.

Nature's pharmacy provides many herbs, extracts, and essences that nourish and support a frayed nervous system. Even the simple act of heading outside to fill your senses with the world of plants has a deeply relaxing, soothing effect on your nerves and psyche.

The Effect of Stress on Adrenal Health

Chronic stress can affect your adrenal glands. The word *adrenal* is Latin for "on the kidneys." The adrenal glands sit directly on top of the kidneys and produce fluids that enable the kidneys to do their job. Thirty-two known hormones are released from the adrenal glands, including adrenaline (a.k.a. epinephrine and noradrenalin or norepinephrine), cortisol, and DHEA. The outer cortex of each adrenal gland secretes corticosteroids, which are made from cholesterol and sex hormones. If the adrenals are constantly on alert due to a stressful lifestyle, they are also constantly producing stress hormones, keeping us in a constant state of fight or flight. In this state, the adrenals can easily become exhausted and depleted.

Signs of adrenal fatigue include recurrent infection, hypoglycemia, fatigue, insomnia, and lower back pain. Without strong adrenals, low testosterone will occur.

Good to Know!

One low-tech way to assess how your adrenal glands are functioning is to bend over and touch your toes. Dizziness when you return to standing may be a sign of weakened adrenal glands. In what is known as tongue diagnosis, a person's tongue may go in and out when they are trying to hold it out, and this is another sign of adrenal fatigue.

Nutritional Therapy

You are what you eat, especially when it comes to handling stress. Eating a naturally colorful whole-food diet that includes organic vegetables, fruits, legumes, nuts, seeds, and oils provides the nutrients, fiber, and phytochemicals you need to improve your defenses against stress. Choosing organic helps you avoid toxic chemicals that may be harmful to mental and emotional health issues as well as the health of our planet.

Eat small, frequent meals, and choose warm, nourishing foods that are high in protein and complex carbohydrates, which help keep blood sugar on an even keel as well as providing important B vitamins. Oatmeal and yogurt are good choices; they are easy to digest and rich in calming calcium. Other good stress-soothing foods include almonds, raisins, and sunflower seeds. Onions contain tension-relieving prostaglandins. Hemp seed and chia seeds provide brain-nourishing omega-3 fatty acids.

Skip This!

Foods that will increase the negative effects of stress include alcohol, caffeinated beverages, fruit juices, sugar, and anything you are allergic to.

Also avoid toxins in the environment, which can stress your nervous system; they include many cleaning products (detergents, fabric softeners, spray cleaners, floor cleaners, etc.) and personal-care supplies (shampoos, other hair products, sunscreens, lotions, perfumes, etc.) Often natural food stores offer options that are gentler for the body, mind, and planet.

Nourishing the Adrenals

The adrenal glands (as well as the kidneys) benefit from mineral-rich black foods such as black sesame seeds, black rice, black quinoa, seaweeds, and chia and sunflower seeds. Avocados, bananas, cantaloupe, peaches, potatoes, chicken, salmon, and tuna are also good tonic food for the adrenals and kidneys. Be sure to get enough protein.

Skip This!

Coffee stimulates the production of adrenaline, our "fight-or-flight hormone." Excessive coffee consumption can lead to adrenal exhaustion, and excessive adrenaline production can cause lactic acid buildup, which can cause an achy feeling.

Supplements for Well-Being

Stress depletes the body's reserves of vitamins and minerals; using supplements during stressful periods will help you reverse the depletion. Consider a vitamin B complex and vitamin C to replenish the water-soluble nutrients. They not only nourish the nervous system but also give you the energy needed to deal with life's problems. Calcium and magnesium help ease tension and irritability. Chromium can help balance blood sugar. Our requirements for these nutrients are increased during difficult times.

You might also consider supplementing with phosphatidylserine, which reduces cortisol levels, thereby taking stress off the adrenal glands.

Healing Herbs

Many soothing, stress-relieving herbs make wonderful teas. Brewing a cup of tea is a good way to slow down, and taking the time to savor a cup of soothing tea is a wonderful way to nourish your nerves. It can give you time to reflect on your day and what's next and how best to handle it. As you drink health-giving teas, inhaling their aromatic virtues, think healing thoughts, like "I am enough" and "All is well in my life now."

Calming herbal baths can provide centering and relaxation if you feel stressed. Put a handful of fresh or dried herbs into a cloth bag (a sock that's lost its mate works just as well), tie it up, and throw it into the tub as it is filling with hot water. You can also add eight to ten drops of your favorite essential oil to the bath once it's full. Get in, inhale the aroma, and feel yourself relax.

The following herbs can be used as tea, tincture, or capsules to soothe stress.

- **Ashwagandha:** Builds chi, helps lower cortisol levels, and helps the adrenals recover from stress.

- **Bacopa:** A nonstimulating adaptogen (it helps the body acclimate to stressful situations).

- **Burdock root:** Improves the function of most organs, including cleansing and nourishing the kidneys and adrenals.

- **California poppy:** A skeletal relaxant that encourages restoration of the nervous system.

- **Catnip:** A nerve tonic that "takes the edge off," as the saying goes.

- **Chamomile:** Tones the nervous system.

- **Eleuthero:** Nourishes the adrenals and is an adaptogen and chi tonic.

- **Ginseng:** Helps the body adapt to stress.

- **Hawthorn:** Calms the spirit and increases circulation to the brain.

- **Hops:** Contains lupulin, a strong but safe and reliable sedative.

- **Kava kava:** Relaxes the muscles without blocking nerve signals and calms physical tension without numbing mental processes.

- **Lemon balm:** Its volatile oils help protect the cerebrum from excessive external stimuli.

- **Licorice:** Relieves adrenal deficiency and exhaustion.

🍃 **Linden:** Calms the nerves and promotes rest.

🍃 **Oatstraw:** Relaxes the nerves and strengthens the nervous system.

🍃 **Passionflower:** Quiets the central nervous system and slows the breakdown of the neurotransmitters serotonin and norepinephrine.

🍃 **Schisandra berry:** An adaptogen and kidney tonic that is rejuvenative and restorative to our entire system, including the adrenals.

🍃 **Skullcap:** Calms and strengthens the nerves, relaxes spasms, relieves pain, and promotes rest.

🍃 **Turmeric:** An antioxidant that nourishes the body's cortisol (a stress hormone) receptor sites.

🍃 **Valerian:** A strong central nervous system relaxant.

🍃 **Wild lettuce:** Calms the nervous system, aids sleep, and relieves pain.

🍃 **Wild oat:** Rich in soothing and nourishing minerals.

🍃 **Wood betony:** Relaxes and strengthens the nerves and relieves pain.

Aromatherapy

Many essential oils have stress-relieving effects. To maximize their effects, use them in combination with other destressing practices, like in warm baths or in the oil used for massage oil. Massage any of the adrenal-nourishing essential oils (diluted in a carrier oil, see page 212 for instructions) over the kidneys and adrenal glands. If you had just one one oil with you all the time, we suggest lavender—it is readily available, pleasant to most, calming, inexpensive, and enjoyed by most people.

Essential Oils to Relieve Stress

Anise	Lemon
Basil	Lemon balm
Bay laurel	Marjoram
Bergamot	Neroli
Cardamom	Nutmeg
Chamomile	Orange
Clary sage	Peppermint
Cypress	Pine
Fennel	Rose
Frankincense	Rosewood
Geranium	Sage
Ginger	Sandalwood
Helichrysum	Spearmint
Jasmine	Tangerine
Juniper	Thyme
Lavender	Ylang-ylang

Essential Oils to Nourish the Adrenals

Basil	Pine
Fir	Rosemary
Juniper	Sage

Mind-Body Therapies and Practices

Many, or even most, forms of mind-body therapies have stress-reducing benefits. Visualization, peaceful mantras (ommmm), yantras (sacred geometry art), and prayer calm the spirit. Biofeedback, hypnosis, guided imagery, and sound healing can all be effective therapies to explore in overcoming stress and anxiety. Explore these options, and all the others available to you, to see which work best for you.

Here, we'll look at a few therapies and practices that are easy to tackle on your own.

Acupressure

Acupressure is easy to do, can be done to oneself, does not involve needles, and provides instant results. Apply pressure to the following points three times, for ten seconds each time, several times a day for general stress or use to calm yourself in stressful situations.

- ▸ Press the point 1½ inches below the navel.
- ▸ Press right below and on the inside corner of the fingernail of the middle finger.
- ▸ Press directly below the inside corner of the nail of the pinkie finger.
- ▸ Place four fingers into the hollow at the base of the skull. Pushing firmly, massage slowly in a circular motion for three minutes.
- ▸ Apply pressure between the first, second, and third thoracic vertebrae.
- ▸ Press the point on top of the hand in the hollow between the thumb and forefinger (LI 4).
- ▸ Press the point where the skull meets the neck on either side of the spine (UB 10).
- ▸ Press the third eye point (Yin Tang)
- ▸ Press directly in the hollow next to the bone on the crease of the wrist in line with the pinkie (HT 7)

The Relaxation Response

The relaxation response is the natural let-down after the fight-or-flight response: Breathing and heart rate slow, muscles relax, and our nervous system returns to a normal level of alertness. With chronic stress, we lose the relaxation response—we simply don't relax. So one powerful way to counter the effects of chronic stress is to intentionally trigger that process of relaxation.

Regular practice of the relaxation response—a concept pioneered by Dr. Herbert Benson at the Benson-Henry Institute for Mind Body Medicine at Massachusetts General Hospital in Boston—has been shown reduce levels of cortisol and epinephrine, feelings of anxiety, and other symptoms of chronic stress. You can elicit the relaxation response in many different ways, including progressive muscle relaxation, diaphragmatic breathing, repetitive prayer, visualization, and guided imagery. Which method to use depends only on what works for you. Let's look at progressive muscle relaxation, a simple technique of bringing your attention to each body part, tightening the muscles there, then relaxing.

Progressive Muscle Relaxation

For this step-by-step, we combine progressive muscle relaxation with a mantra—a word or phrase you repeat to yourself to focus your mental energy, which clears mental clutter, reduces stimulation in the emotional center of the brain, and helps you feel calmer.

Start by doing this full exercise for ten minutes, twice a day, and work up to twenty. The more you practice the relaxation response, the better you will feel.

- *Sit or lie down in a quiet place.*
- *Take a deep breath in, noticing your lungs and abdomen filling with air.*
- *Then breathe out, relaxing your core, and visualizing all tension leaving your body with your breath.*
- *Repeat a few times.*
- *Tighten the muscles of your forehead by raising your eyebrows as high as you can. Hold for a few seconds, then release. Breathe, feeling the tension leaving your forehead.*
- *Now tighten the muscles of your eyes, squeezing them closed. Hold for a few seconds, then release. Breathe, appreciating the relaxation of your eye muscles.*
- *Continue in this way, from head to toe, progressively tightening and then relaxing all the muscles of your body.*
- *When you're done, focus on repeating a mantra—a word*

or phrase—silently to yourself. When other thoughts arise, notice them, but do not engage; detach and let them go.

Yoga Nidra

Yoga nidra, or yogic sleep, is the easiest yoga you'll ever practice, since it's done while you are sitting or lying down. It's also deeply relaxing and healing. You'll follow a guide, whether in person or via a recording, who will lead you through a meditation that helps you access the *koshas,* or states of mind and body that enhance psychological, physical, and spiritual health and well-being. These koshas include the physical body of sensation and the bodies of breath and energy, feelings and emotions, thoughts, and joy.

Research conducted at Stanford University, Walter Reed National Military Medical Center, Ohio State University, and other institutions has proved yoga nidra's effectiveness in improving health. A 2007 study in the journal *Psycho-Oncology* showed that guided imagery like the kind used in yoga nidra helps relieve anxiety, and research is ongoing on the effects of yoga nidra on post-traumatic stress syndrome.

The more you practice yoga nidra, the more you'll experience its benefits. Generally, it takes fifteen to forty-five minutes, every day or second day (but not after a meal). Yoga teacher Jennifer Reis's Divine Sleep yoga nidra guided meditations and teacher trainings are excellent; you can find them online.

Forest Bathing

Ancient traditions and current research have shown that forest bathing, known in Japan as *shinrin-yoku,* helps lower cortisol levels and gets you out of the fight-or-flight mode. Forest bathing is much what it sounds like: going to the forest and soaking up the sights, sounds, and scents found there. The practice can be as simple as taking a walk in the woods. Research published in the *International Journal of Environmental Health Research,* among other places, shows the clear benefits of this sort of "green exercise" on blood pressure, self-esteem, and mood.

One reason forest bathing may be so powerful is the presence of negative ions—molecules in the air that carry an electrical charge. Negative ions are generated by many plants as part of their natural growth cycle. They're also formed by water crashing into itself, such as you might find at a waterfall, in a fast-moving stream, or at the beach. Forest air tends to be full of them, and they have been shown to lower oxidative stress and influence the inflammatory compounds in the body that affect your mood. (You can tap into this soothing effect at home with a desktop fountain.)

Gardening

If you have a green thumb, or would like to, spending time in the garden is one of the most enjoyable and effective ways to reduce stress. Plants reduce blood pressure, increase concentration and productivity, and help recovery from illness. A study done at Utsunomiya University in Japan showed that working with plants helps reduce fatigue and bring calm. The participants were in one of three groups: filling pots with soil, transplanting nonflowering pansy plants, or transplanting flowering plants. Those who worked with the flowering plants had more positive results than those who worked with the nonflowering plants.

Start simply by just looking at plants—outside, inside, wherever you are. Enjoy the view out your window, or set a vase of flowers on your table. Try easy-care houseplants—your local gardening center should be able to give you recommendations. Then, in spring, move outside to garden. Remember, gardening is an affirmation for a fruitful future!

If you lack outdoor space, try container gardening. The EarthBox, a self-watering container garden system, provides an easy way to grow flowers or vegetables; you can find it online. You can also become a member of a community garden in your town. You can even learn to harvest and eat weeds—many are wildly nutritious!

Find Peace with a Slow Hobby

Slow hobbies such as knitting, painting, sculpting, sketching, crocheting, or quilting have a meditative quality that can reduce stress and help you relax, along with improving focus and concentration. According to recent Craft Yarn Council research, 64 percent of knitters and crocheters use these crafts to help them reduce stress and relax. Studies show that these hobbies help lower heart rate and blood pressure. How do you find the right slow hobby for you? Choose something you really enjoy to put this remedy into practice. Visit a craft store and see what looks fun. There even may be something you enjoyed doing as a child that you can enjoy doing now.

Write It Down

Keeping a journal of your daily experiences can help you learn what triggers you and what you need to change in order to feel more peaceful. Just putting pen to paper and releasing your troubles is therapeutic. Try this exercise to get started.

☞ Get the Stress Out of Your Head

1. Make two lists: one of the stresses in your life you can change, the other of the stresses you can't.
2. Rate them on a scale of one to ten, with ten being the highest. Take a moment to acknowledge and reflect on each stressor and the effect it has on you.
3. For the stresses you can change, write down possible solutions or actions. It could be as simple as asking for help, initiating a new daily habit, or reasearching a countermeasure.
4. For the stresses you can't change, write down possible actions you could take—making a small donation to a cause, writing a letter to the editor, joining a group that is taking action. Or, if none of these are possible, perhaps journal an acknowledgment that this stressor is outside of your con-

trol but what you can control is how you react to it. Then go back to possible solutions regarding your actions and reactions.

5. Come back to this exercise whenever stresses feel like they are mounting again!

Another trick is to keep a journal-like to-do list. When your brain starts to cycle through all the many tasks and responsibilities on your plate, in a seemingly endless loop, turn to your list. Write down what you need to do, then let it go from your thoughts. This practice not only helps you avoid forgetting what needs to be done but also avoids feelings of overwhelm. "If you think it, ink it!"

Practical Tips to Reduce Stress

Try these tips to reduce stress and bring serenity to your days.

Exercise. Exercise improves respiration and circulation, sends nutrients to the cells, stimulates endorphin production, and flushes out stress.

Give yourself a massage. Focus on your hands, face, and feet. Or try massage therapy—it's a great stress reliever.

Reach out to someone. Hug your child, love your mate, lend a hand to a friend in need, or pet your cat or dog.

Breathe more deeply and slowly. Oxygen nourishes the brain. Alternate nostril breathing is an excellent technique to create a balance in both hemispheres of the brain.

Slow down. Slow your eating, talking, walking, and driving. Do whatever you need to do, but do it more slowly. Enunciate. Even speaking more calmly can have a calming effect.

Wear blue and green. These colors are relaxing and calming. Avoid excess yellow, as it contributes to anxiety. Wear comfortable clothing that allows your skin to breathe and freedom of movement.

Try a relaxing bath. Light a candle; add a few drops of the stress-relieving essential oils mentioned earlier in this chapter. Soak and enjoy. When you're done, let the water run down the drain as you visualize all your stress going with it.

Listen to calming, contemplative music.

Prepare for tomorrow. Pull together everything you need to get started the next day—your clothes, paperwork, schedule, and perhaps lunch—the night before, rather than starting your morning in a frenzy.

Get up early. In the morning, get out of bed fifteen minutes earlier than you have to in order to allow time to take care of what's needed calmly.

Keep a to-do list and a calendar. Rather than letting your mind carry around all the logistical details of your life, write it down! Use a calendar or scheduling app, take notes on paper or in your phone—do what works best for you. (Brigitte lives by her *Law of Attraction Planner* book to keep track of appointments and commitments, and always has it by her side.)

Get it over with. Take care of unpleasant or difficult tasks early in the day, so the rest of the time can be spent more easily.

Learn to say no. You don't have to do everything asked of you. Practice saying, "No," or at least, "I'll think about it."

Get rid of clutter in your life. Clutter causes confusion and stress.

Practice visualization. There are guided versions available where you close your eyes and visualize yourself . . . floating on a cloud, lying by a trickling brook, or whatever experience you wish. Visit these tranquil places in your mind. (Chrystle particularly loves Creative Visualization Meditations by Shakti Gawain to help relax, create an inner sanctuary, and access intuition.)

Learn a craft. Playing with clay is especially stress relieving, and creating things of beauty is great for self-esteem.

Get a set of Chinese hand balls. Learn to use them to give the mind a focus and the body repetitive movement to create calm.

Be prepared . . . to wait. For those times when you find yourself waiting—in line, at school pickup, on hold—have something to do so you don't have to feel like you are wasting time. It could be something to read, a relaxation technique to practice, knitting, or anything that is simple to bring along and easy to do quickly or jump in and out of.

Smile. Relaxing your face helps the rest of your body as well as putting at ease those around you.

Talk to a sympathetic listener.

Enlist the help of others. Delegate. You don't have to do everything yourself.

Read books that are uplifting to you. Be careful where you put your consciousness. (Maybe try *The Urantia Book,* the Bible, or Tao Te Ching.)

Spend time basking in the beauty of nature. Go outside and look at the sky. Sit by a stream. Take a walk in the woods.

Watch fish in an aquarium.

Every day, do something you really enjoy.

Act like a kid. Throw a Frisbee. Read fairy tales. Undertake imaginative adventures.

Do something for someone less fortunate than you.

Take things one at a time.

Pray for guidance.

Meditate.

Take a short nap when you can. Use earplugs or a white noise machine to ensure quiet.

Don't take on what's not yours. Don't assume that the success or failure of your children, your partner, your parents is entirely the result of your influence.

Spend quality time with people you care about.

Have more fun.

Have some alone time every day.

Remember that you don't need to be perfect.

Get in touch with an old friend.

Plan something to look forward to.

Do what you can to change a stressful situation.

Use your voice to speak more affirmatively. For example, saying "I am going to figure this out" is less stress-inducing than repeating "I am doomed."

Count your blessings.

The most effective way to deal with stress is to focus on self-care. Taking small actions every day will help you defuse stress when it arises, enabling you to return to calm more easily. Think of it as depositing serenity into your well-being bank. If you don't make regular deposits, you won't have the peace of mind that you need to counterbalance stressful situations.

So you don't feel overwhelmed, begin by working to incorporate just one of the stress-reducing strategies described in this chapter into your regular routine, whether it's taking fifteen minutes each day for yoga, adding a new nourishing food to your diet, drinking a daily cup of herbal tea, or journaling about how you feel.

Most importantly, be patient with yourself as you adopt the practices that work best for you. Over time, you will find that you feel calmer, less stressed, and more in control of your emotions, your days, and your life.

2
Anxiety

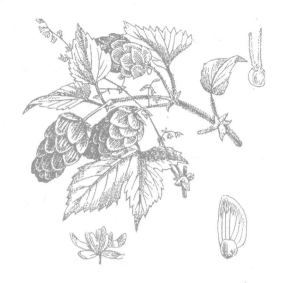

Do not anticipate trouble, or worry about what may never happen. Keep in the sunlight.

BENJAMIN FRANKLIN

Making room for more joy and happiness in your life means learning how to manage uncomfortable emotions like anxiety more effectively. Natural remedies and practices can help you deal with and soothe your anxiety and clear the way for a more peaceful, well-balanced you.

What Is Anxiety?

The word *anxiety* comes from the Latin *angustia,* meaning "narrowness, restriction, or difficulty." It's an apt description, because when we feel fearful, our world constricts. Anxiety can be a warning of impending pain or potential danger, triggering alertness—a useful quality, as this planet can be a perilous place. It can also be provoked by fear (of the known or unknown) and can occur when we are out of harmony within ourselves or with the people and things around us.

In reality, anxiety is unrelated to any real, imminent danger. It is an overreaction of the autonomic nervous system, where the flight-or-fight mechanism is activated and exaggerated. When this happens the stress hormones adrenaline and cortisol are released to help us deal with danger, real or imagined.

Causes

Heredity, trauma (including while in utero), difficult birth or childhood, blood sugar imbalances, glandular disorders, respiratory disorders, digestive disorders, major stress, physical illness, and medication can all contribute to anxiety. Research indicates that a biochemical imbalance in the amygdala (the brain's alarm center, located in the emotional center of the brain) can cause this psychological imbalance. It's not unusual to suffer from anxiety *and* depression.

Excessive copper in the body (from copper pipes or cookware) can be a contributing factor in anxiety. Yeast overgrowth can contribute to anxiety, and anxiety contributes to yeast overgrowth. In ayurvedic medicine, anxiety is considered an imbalance of *vata,* the air element.

Symptoms

Anxiety can feel like you've had way too much coffee, like a swarm of bees is buzzing around you, or like an electrical charge is running throughout your body. Regardless, it's very uncomfortable! Other symptoms can include clammy hands, rapid heartbeat, muscle tension, nausea, stomach distress, and shallow, rapid breathing resulting in excessive carbon dioxide, which can make you feel light-headed, dizzy, numb, tingly, or sweaty; you may experience chest pain.

Long-Term Effects

Chronic anxiety can increase the risk of heart attack, precipitate an asthma attack, worsen diabetes, and weaken immunity, making us more susceptible to cancer as well as colds, flus, and herpes outbreaks.

Different Types of Anxiety

Anxiety manifests in many different ways. If you always feel fearful, no matter what is actually happening, you might have generalized anxiety disorder. Having a panic disorder means you experience sudden attacks of severe anxiety, which are very frightening and can make you feel out of control. The attacks are brief, lasting only a few minutes, but can be misidentified as a heart attack since you can experience heart palpitations, shortness of breath, and dizziness. Once you have an attack, you may begin to avoid situations that you think provoke them.

Obsessive-compulsive disorder (OCD) is another form of anxiety disorder. If you have OCD, you tend to have obsessive thoughts or actions, like going over your to-do list twenty times, washing your hands repeatedly, or checking and rechecking to make sure a door is locked, in a false belief that it will keep bad things from happening.

Phobias, too, are anxiety disorders, in this case causing fear of subjects ranging from heights to flying to snakes and more.

Good to Know!
Common Phobias

- Acrophobia: fear of heights
- Agoraphobia: fear of open or crowded places, of leaving one's home, of being trapped
- Arachnophobia: fear of spiders
- Chionophobia: fear of snow
- Claustrophobia: fear of closed spaces
- Cynophobia: fear of dogs
- Kathisophobia: fear of sitting down
- Musophobia: fear of mice
- Ophidiophobia: fear of snakes

There are many natural remedies that can help calm and even prevent anxiety. Some of these natural remedies are becoming more well-known but others may be new to you. We encourage you to explore the remedies that most resonate with you.

Nutritional Therapy

Feeding the brain and the central nervous system with the right foods can help soothe anxiety. The best antianxiety diet is one that keeps your blood sugar at a steady level morning, noon, and night, because symptoms may worsen when your blood sugar dips. This means choosing lean proteins, whole grains, veggies, and fruit and nixing refined sugars and starches.

Anxiety is more likely to occur when blood sugar is low. The most important thing is to avoid getting too hungry. You may do best "grazing" all day long, eating four to six small meals and snacks; carry nuts, cheese, crackers, sunflower seeds, or pumpkin seeds with you each day.

Skip This!

As best you can, avoid coffee, excitotoxins such as MSG (monosodium glutamate), artificial sweeteners, stimulants, asthma medications, decongestants, and antidepressants. All drugs and alcohol can trigger anxiety, rev you up, and put your body into panic-alert overtime.

Also avoid any foods you might be allergic to, as they can cause increased pulse, thus provoking a feeling of anxiety and potentially even triggering a panic attack. If necessary, keep a food diary to determine which foods bother you the most.

Other foods to focus on include those that have high levels of calming calcium, like oatmeal and yogurt. Lettuce also helps calm anxiety. Nutrient-dense, grounding foods such as buckwheat, chia, millet, black quinoa, black rice, black sesame seeds, sea vegetables, sweet potatoes, and winter squash are also helpful.

Good to Know!

Unstable blood sugar levels can lead to depression and anxiety. In fact, a hypoglycemic (low blood sugar) reaction mimics the physiological symptoms of a panic attack. This is why it's so important to keep your blood sugar on an even keel instead of a sugar-powered roller coaster. Carry a few Brazil nuts with you for a lightweight, yet filling snack.

Mother Nature's News

A 2011 study published in *Brain, Behavior, and Immunity* showed that people who took fish oil supplements had a 20 percent reduction in anxiety and a significant reduction in inflammation. If you want to try this supplement as a way to alleviate anxiety, be sure to find a high-quality, pure fish oil supplement that has been tested by a third party to avoid heavy metals like mercury, contaminants, and other toxins.

Fish oil is helpful primarily as a source of omega-3 fatty acids. There are also vegan sources of omega-3s, including blue-green algae, chia seeds, hemp seeds, and walnuts; see page 306 for more sources.

Supplements for Well-Being

Daily supplementation of calcium, magnesium, and B complex can contribute to calming anxiety. You can also supplement with inositol, a compound that works as a cell messenger for our nervous system. Inositol's effect is similar to that of the benzodiazepine drug Librium (chlordiazepoxide); it can help calm panic and improves symptoms of OCD. Another option is 5-HTP (5-hydroxytryptophan), preferably taken between meals, which may be effective against anxiety disorders.

Many people suffering from anxiety have low levels of GABA (gamma-aminobutyric acid), a neurotransmitter that helps neurons "talk" to each other and protects the brain from overstimulation. You can take a GABA supplement (preferably sublingually), or try passionflower, which boosts GABA levels. DMAE (dimethylethanolamine) is another option; naturally present in fish and sardines, this compound protects cellular membranes and transports readily across the bloodbrain barrier to calm anxiety.

Amino acids are important when it comes to calming the nervous system and easing anxiety. Glycine quiets cells in the spinal cord, brain stem, and central nervous system. Taurine suppresses the release of overexciting neurotransmitters like norepinephrine. Histidine calms beta waves and promotes more relaxing alpha waves. Methionine helps reduce histamine levels, which are often elevated in people with OCD. You can also find supplements that include combinations of amino acids.

Healing Herbs

You've probably heard of kava kava, a plant native to the South Pacific, whose extract has been used for thousands of years in rituals and ceremonies and as a social drink. The eighteenth-century British explorer Captain James Cook gave it its Latin name, *Piper methysticum,* meaning "intoxicating pepper." The majority of evidence shows that certain kava extracts (standardized to 70 percent kavalactones) can lower anxiety and may be as effective as low-dose benzodiazepines in relieving anxiety.

As noted, passionflower increases levels of GABA. A small study published in the *Journal of Clinical Pharmacy and Therapeutics* in 2001 showed that passionflower is as effective as oxazepam (brand name Serax, a medication used to ease anxiety disorders) for treating generalized anxiety disorder, without any of the side effects.

Adaptogens, which help the body adapt to stress, can be very helpful in relieving anxiety. Try ashwagandha, eleuthero, ginkgo, ginseng, and reishi, all of which can help calm or energize depending on what the body needs.

Other helpful herbs include the following:

- **California poppy:** Cooling and calming and soothes the emotional body.

- **Hawthorn:** Nourishes the physical and emotional heart.

- **Wild lettuce extract:** Helps calm generalized anxiety

- **Wild oat:** Helps calm acute anxiety.

Choose soothing herbal teas such as catnip, chamomile, hawthorn, lemon balm, oatstraw, passionflower, or reishi mushroom. Hops and valerian calm anxiety but don't taste pleasant, so try a tincture or capsules instead. When you're feeling especially anxious, brew a cup of herbal tea, take one to three dropperfuls of tincture, or take an herbal capsule three times daily between meals.

!

Cure Caution

Herbs like kava kava can help ease anxiety, but if you are already taking prescription medication for your condition, check with your doctor before adding any natural remedies for anxiety.

Homeopathy

Homeopathic remedies are a safe and gentle way to ease anxiety. Read through the descriptions for each cure and see which one sounds most like your situation, then try it. Usually three to four pellets are placed under the tongue to dissolve.

- **Aconitum napellus:** For sudden stress, or for stress after a danger such as earthquake, tornado, or other natural disaster.

- **Argentum nitricum:** For performance anxiety or fear of the unknown.

- **Arsenicum album:** For those always in motion, calms anxiety

- **Calcarea carbonica:** For anxiety about your mental and physical health, catching infections, and misfortune. For the person who is overworked and easily discouraged.

- **Coffea cruda:** For paralyzing anxiety preceding an event such as flying or public speaking.

- **Gelsemium:** For anxiety over exams and public speaking; for stage fright.

- **Ignatia:** For acute anxiety after a breakup or death of a loved one. For the person who attempts to hold back emotions but cannot, perhaps alternately sobbing and laughing.

- **Kali phosphoricum:** For the person who is easily startled, overexcited, or fearful of having a nervous breakdown.

- **Lachesis:** For anxiety that you're being conspired against and nighttime anxiety.

- **Lycopodium:** For anxiety in social situations. For the person who is overly concerned with what people think of them.

- **Natrum muriaticum:** For the person who stoicly hides anxiety, who rarely cries in front of others, refuses sympathy, but will sob when left alone.

- **Passiflora incarnata:** For general anxiety and obsessive thoughts.

- **Silica:** For anxiety about exams, public speaking, and interviews. For the person who is shy yet strong-willed.

Flower Essences

Flower essences can help balance negative emotions, freeing the body's energy to heal itself.

- **Agrimony:** Calms deep-seated anxiety and restlessness, helping one feel more grounded.

- **Aspen:** For fear and anxiety when you don't really know what is the cause. Promotes a sense of calm and security.

- **Heather:** For those who are constantly obsessed with small problems and need to tell everyone about them.

- **Larch:** Restores well-being in one who feels constant low-level anxiety like a persistent hum.

- **Mimulus:** For worry that things will not work out, misfortune will occur, and suffering will result. For anxiety about money and health. Helps to put things into perspective.

- **Rescue Remedy:** For general anxiety and to reduce stress and tension.

- **White Chestnut:** For persistent unwanted thoughts, preoccupation, insomnia, or nervous worry.

Keep flower essences on hand in convenient places, such as in your bag, your desk, and the glove compartment of your car, and use them when you feel anxiety start to come on. Two drops under the tongue is all it takes. You could also add a few drops of the remedy to a glass of water and sip it slowly. If you are sensitive to the alcohol in flower essences, apply the remedies externally to your wrists and/or temples or purchase one of the new non-alcohol tinctures.

Aromatherapy

Aromatherapy is one of the quickest and most effective ways to soothe anxiety. The nasal cavities are in very close proximity to the brain, linking our sense of smell and the limbic or emotional center of the brain. And, of course, breathing deeply itself has a quick positive effect.

If you aren't sure which essential oils work best for you, try several different types and see how you react. Then, when you are feeling anxious, put three or four drops on a tissue and inhale deeply. Or take five to ten deep inhalations right from the bottle! It saves paper. Brigitte likes to put two drops in the palm of her hands, rub them together, lift to her face and take several deep inhalations to immediately open different neural pathways. Rather than traveling down Freak Out Freeway, just take a stroll down Lavender Lane. You can also put essential oils in a diffuser to fill any room with an anxiety-reducing aroma. Have some essential oils to use with you everywhere: desk, bag, first aid kit, and so on.

Good choices include:

Basil	Lemon balm
Bergamot	Marjoram
Cedarwood	Myrrh
Chamomile	Neroli
Clary sage	Orange
Cypress	Petitgrain
Geranium	Rose
Hyssop	Rosemary
Jasmine	Sandalwood
Juniper	Thyme
Lavender	Ylang-ylang

Good to Know!

Lavender is easy to grow and care for. Harvest the flowers, make them into a sachet, and place it near your pillow when sleeping to reduce anxiety and induce sleep.

Mind-Body Therapies and Practices

Just as we may spend time working on our physique with exercise, there are many practices available that can augment all that we do for a healthier body and mind. Taking time out for self-care and self-love is part of the healing journey. Anything we can do that gets us to slow down, be present, and make wise decisions can help us calm anxiety.

☞ Take Control When Panic Attacks

- *When a panic attack occurs, sit down, keeping your knees uncrossed.*
- *Breathe slowly.*
- *Put your hands firmly on the surface in front of you—a table, the arms of your chair, the floor—and say "STOP" aloud.*
- *Work on keeping your body relaxed and breathing slow. Remember that however panicked you are, this feeling will pass and not harm you.*
- *Try to focus on something else. Say a comforting prayer or a sacred chant or mantra, or count backward from 100 by threes. Or try focusing on a still object in the room, observing it so closely that you lose yourself in its details. Another technique is to grab an object, such as an orange, and with your hands in front of your chest, switch the orange from hand to hand in a gentle sweeping motion to balance the brain's hemispheres. Continue the technique of your choice until you feel calm.*
- *Take up to five deep inhalations from a bottle of lavender essential oil in each nostril.*
- *Afterward, when you are calm, give the episode a rating of 1 to 10, 10 being extreme panic. Then you can ask yourself what the attack was trying to protect you from. Write about your answers and feelings. Visualize how you want things to go in your life and write about it.*

Acupressure

Gently press or rub the space between the eyebrows in the center of the forehead to help calm anxiety and thus the *shen* (spirit). Apply pressure to the center of the left upper palm, between the base of the middle and ring fingers, with the right hand firmly for one minute to calm anxiety. Another technique is to hold the thumb of one hand with the other to calm and ground yourself. Holding your toes, especially the middle toe, helps bring energy down from the head and ground it. Generally you can apply pressure to the these points three times, for ten seconds each time, several times a day or repeat as needed.

Good to Know!

According to the principles of traditional Chinese medicine, the kidneys correspond to the element of water and govern the bones, teeth, hair on our head, sense of hearing, and emotions of fear and willpower. Keeping the kidneys nourished and warm by dressing warmly can help calm your anxiety and make you feel safe and empowered.

Try, also, wearing the color blue. It's tranquil and soothing to the spirit.

Cognitive Behavioral Therapy

While these natural remedies and techniques can help ease anxiety, see your health care practitioner if anxiety is significantly affecting your day-to-day living. These natural therapies are not a substitute for proper medical care. With more serious disorders like phobias, generalized anxiety disorder, panic attacks, or OCD, you may need a combination of therapy and prescription medication to function more effectively.

One traditional therapy to consider is cognitive behavioral therapy (CBT). This type of therapy is particularly helpful for phobias and is proactive and goal oriented, helping you identify negative behaviors and thought patterns and then change them so they are more positive.

For example, if you have anxiety, you may think, "I am always in danger." A CBT therapist might work with you to challenge that irrational belief and replace it with a more realistic view of reality—for example, "I am safe." Since it's an active process, you'll be encouraged to write down your anxious thoughts and practice new ways of behaving outside of your sessions.

Research shows that CBT is useful for anxiety disorders, helping to change brain functioning and helping you feel calmer. Ultimately, CBT is about taking control of your negative thoughts and changing them to positive ones so you feel happier.

Write It Down

If worry persists, consider taking the last five minutes of every hour to write down what is worrying you so as to identify the problems.

☛ Setting Action Steps

1. Separate the issues causing you anxiety into categories—for example, home, family, work.
2. Next, ask what you can do about each worry right now.
3. If you can take action on a particular problem, break it down into smaller steps. Write them down as a to-do list or in your day planner.
4. Take action, one step at a time.

Another helpful journaling technique is to ask yourself: "What is the worst that can happen?" Write down your answers. Once you know what that is, chances are you'll be able to face the possibilities with more sanity.

You can also use your journal to keep track of the factors that might contribute to anxious feelings or panic attacks. Are there any common denominators, such as a food, place, theme, certain person, or situation?

Make a list of the people and places you typically encounter. Ask which of those feel safe and which don't. Put a mark by all those that feel threatening, and try to limit your exposure to them. Create safe space in your home, in your work space, and with friends and family. See how that makes you feel.

Conscious Media

Anxiety can be driven or exacerbated by media. Where you place your consciousness affects your reality. Most mainstream media is controlled by a few companies who are determined to push their own agenda for power and profits. So, choose what goes into your mind wisely. Overwatching the news, spending too much time and energy on social media, and watching movies and reading books designed to fill us with fear and dread can be very detrimental to our mental and emotional health.

Minimize social media time if it is not serving your highest good. Posts on social media can trigger feelings of anxiety, envy, FOMO (fear of missing out), depression, and even anger. So, turn off notifications and even your phone when possible.

Make it a habit to check in with yourself throughout the day and ask, "Is this book [movie, post, video, etc.] adding to my knowledge, helping me to be a better person, helping me feel more positive, or is it a distraction or desctructive?

Practical Tips for Managing Anxiety

Anxiety is not always easy to manage, but there are some simple, practical steps you can take to keep your emotions from growing beyond your control.

Take action. There's a saying: The antidote to anxiety is action. In other words, when you're feeling worried or anxious about a particular issue, focus on doing something about it. If you can't figure out what to do, brainstorm solutions with a trusted friend.

Unburden. Share your problems with a trusted friend or family member. Tell them what is troubling you. Clear your mind and heart.

Stay busy. Being busy crowds out worry. Active people don't have time to worry!

Prepare. When attending situations that are likely to cause anxiety, go with a friend, avoid sugar and alcohol beforehand, and be sure to take your calming supplements, like your B vitamins, before leaving.

Set boundaries. If you must worry about things, designate one hour of the day to this activity. When that hour is up, you're done!

Accept. If you are feeling anxious but can't take action in that moment, try the Serenity Prayer: God [or whatever force you hold sacred] grant me the serenity to accept the things I cannot change, the courage to change the things I can, and the wisdom to know the difference.

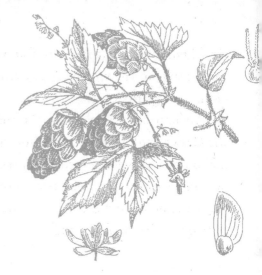

3
Fear

Fear falls before the fortress of faith.

Fear is one way Nature helps protect us from danger and getting into trouble. The moment the body recognizes fear, the amygdala, an almond-shaped gland in our brains, directs a cascade of energy, causing us to be ready for fight or flight. The heart beats faster; adrenals secrete cortisol and adrenaline (a.k.a. epinephrine), heightening our focus and awareness. Blood is shunted to the major muscles and brain. As a result, we may experience coldness in the extremities, uneven breath, high blood pressure, pallor, nausea, sweaty palms, dry mouth, dry vagina, tight chest and muscles, dilated pupils, and trembling.

There are many natural remedies that can support us in facing our fears with more balance. Several natural remedies for fearfulness are aimed at nourishing and balancing the kidneys, as this is the seat of fear in traditional Chinese medicine.

Fear and the Kidneys

According to traditional Chinese medicine, the root of fear is in the kidney water element. Not only can weakness in the kidneys cause fearfulness, but excessive fear can lead to weakness in the kidneys. Kidney yin (fluids) are more a factor in fear, while kidney yang (chi or energy) corresponds to the willpower to overcome fears. Excessive fear causes kidney energy to descend.

An imbalance in the kidneys can manifest emotionally in being withdrawn, unforgiving, and suspicious. Long-term fear can contribute to physical symptoms that may include low back ache, feeling cold, hearing problems, puffiness around the eyes, and sometimes even blue discoloration around the eyes. A deficiency in kidney chi can manifest in frequent dreams of drowning.

Nutritional Therapy

Winter squash and buckwheat are strengthening foods; energetically, they can help courage triumph over fear. And as a general rule, eat warm foods; they are more comforting to the emotion of fear than anything icy cold.

To help prevent fearfulness, avoid foods that stimulate or sensitize the nervous system, like alcohol, caffeine, artificial sweeteners and dyes, and MSG.

In terms of supplements, B-complex vitamins, especially B_1, niacin, and choline, and a calcium-magnesium supplement will help give you the fortitude to face fears. L-glutamine, GABA, and omega-3 fatty acids can also be helpful.

Healing Herbs

Herbs to fortify us against the fear factor include eleuthero, ginseng, kava kava, skullcap, and valerian; try them as tinctures, teas, or capsules. The culinary herb thyme has been traditionally used to give people the courage to speak out. Because parsley is rich in kidney-nourishing chlorophyll, it is excellent to use in liberal amounts in food preparation.

Borage is said give courage, and its beautiful blue flowers were once embroidered on the mantles of knights going off to battle. The flowers are edible; use them to garnish salads and other dishes.

Good to Know!

Borage is an easy to grow annual and it attracts pollinators to your window box or garden.

Chinese Patent Medicine

The Chinese patent formula called Ding Xin Wan, also known as "Calm Heart Pill," calms the shen (spirit) and is used to treat restlessness, fright, and anxiety.

Homeopathy

Homeopathic remedies that help us face fear include:

- **Aconitum napellus:** For acute fear, shock, anxiety, restlessness, and insomnia. For sudden fears due to natural disasters, accidents, and shock. For fear of death. For the person who wakes up frightened, with heart palpitations, who is sensitive to light, noise, and touch.

- **Argentum nitricum:** For the person who fears crowds and is afraid, nervous, and impulsive. For fear that causes diarrhea.

- **Arsenicum album:** For fear of being alone. For the person who is restless, fussy, fastidious, and obsessive; who fears loss of control, illness, and death; who is always in motion.

- **Belladonna:** For fear of animals, dogs, and snakes.

- **Calcarea carbonica:** For children who fear the dark, insects, cats, and dogs. For fear of misfortune, disease, loss of reason, and insanity.

- **Causticum:** For fear of animals.

- **Cinchona:** For fear of animals, especially cats and dogs.

- **Gelsemium:** For fears of exams and public speaking; for stage fright.

- **Ignatia:** For fear of birds. For dread.

- **Kali carbonicum:** For fear of being alone, especially after dark.

- **Lachesis:** For fear of snakes.

- **Lycopodium:** For fear, anxiety, and insecurity. For the person who is nervous in social situations and overly concerned with what people think of them. For fear of animals. For fear of rejection, aging, change, and loss of position.

- **Natrum muriaticum:** For fear of birds, snakes, spiders, and insanity.

- **Nux vomica:** For fear of insanity.

- **Tuberculinum:** For fear of animals, especially cats. For the person who always feels criticized.

- **Phosphorus:** For the person who is tall and thin and excessively sensitive, afraid of the dark, being alone, ghosts, and storms. For the person who has an active imagination.

- **Pulsatilla:** For the person whose fear causes lots of tears. For fear of dogs, snakes, and insanity.

- **Sepia:** For dread.

- **Silicea:** For fear of needles.

Flower Essences

Flower essences can be another avenue for overcoming fear. Some to consider include:

- **Aspen:** For fear of the unknown, including fear of the dark.

🌿 **Cherry Plum:** For fear of mental collapse.

🌿 **Blackberry:** For fear of death. For the person who is lethargic, negative, and fault finding.

🌿 **Garlic:** For the person who is fearful and weak, with low vitality.

🌿 **Larch:** For fear of failure.

🌿 **Mimulus:** For fear of pain, dark, accidents, poverty, being alone, and misfortune.

🌿 **Red Chestnut:** For fear for the safety of others.

🌿 **Rock Rose:** For terror and panic; for hysteria due to accidents and trauma. For nightmares. For the person who is overly concerned with the problems of the world and projects this onto others.

🌿 **Rescue Remedy:** For fear of anything.

Aromatherapy

Essential oils that help calm fear and fortify the nerves can be helpful. Try massaging a few drops of them over the kidneys. Good ones to consider include:

Angelica	Lavender
Basil	Lemon balm
Bergamot	Lemongrass
Cedarwood	Neroli
Chamomile	Orange
Clary sage	Patchouli
Coriander	Pine
Cypress	Rose
Fennel	Rosewood
Fir	Sandalwood
Frankincense	Spruce

Geranium	Thyme
Hyssop	Vanilla
Jasmine	Vetiver
Juniper	Ylang-ylang

Mind-Body Therapies and Practices

An acupressure point that can help calm fear is the bony spot right below the center of the eye, nearest the lower eyelid. Press here for thirty seconds while imagining the fear. Then tap on the outside of each of your second toes (next to the big toe) for thirty seconds, while continuing to imagine what you are afraid of.

Consider taking up t'ai chi and qigong; both help strengthen the kidneys. If you practice yoga, try the Lion pose, which can help dispel fear.

Practice meditation and visualization techniques to learn more control over your mind. Practice deep, slow, rhythmic breathing so your brain can benefit from the calming properties of sufficient oxygen as well as to help direct the mind.

When fearfulness spins up to a moment of true fright, find quiet space and warmth. Curling up in a fetal position can help relieve the feeling. Try applying a hot water bottle over the kidneys and on the bottom of your feet, as fear is considered a cold condition.

To ward off such episodes, try wearing and visualizing the color magenta, which helps strengthen the emotions against fear as well as balance the kidneys.

The best time to face your fears is when you first notice there is a problem. Otherwise, they may grow over time and become more unmanageable. But please, take the process slowly. Focus on the step you are on, rather than the next step. These guidelines can help:

☞ Facing Fears

1. *Recognize what you are avoiding. What does your fear protect you from? How does it keep you stuck?*

2. *Gradually integrate your fear by degrees, starting in an environment that makes you feel safe. For example, if you have a fear of crowds, start by going to a small party of close friends before attending a festival.*

3. *Give each fearful episode a rating on a scale of one to ten—one being the least fearful and ten the most fearful. As you gradually increase exposure, check in with where you land on that scale each time.*

4. *Reward yourself for being brave with something that feels nourishing to you—reading a good book, an aromatherapy bath, visiting a friend, a cup of chamomile tea.*

Defusing Fear of Public Speaking

Fearfulness around public speaking is very common. Try these tips to defuse your fear:

▸ Reframe: See the event as exciting rather than frightening.

▸ Prepare: Practice—a lot! Research your subject well. Prepare notes you can refer to in order to trigger your memory and keep you on track.

▸ Know your audience: There's no point in addressing a group of teenagers the same way you would address a group of lawyers. Let go of the outcome but visualize success.

▸ Know the space: If you're not familiar with the space where you'll be speaking, see if you can get a look at it ahead of time. Find out whether you will use a microphone.

▸ Support your nerves: Take some tryptophan or Rescue Remedy an hour beforehand.

▸ Support your voice: Drink something warm before speaking to open your voice. Honey and lemon in hot water is excellent.

▸ Carry something: Some people find that they feel more confident if they can hold something (e.g., a newspaper, umbrella, magic crystal) while they are speaking.

▸ Ground yourself: Yawn several times before addressing a group (privately, of course)—yawning bring more oxygen into the body, thus improving alertness. Slow your breathing, which calms your heart and helps you speak at a comfortable pace. Put your feet firmly on the floor and visualize being grounded and breathing up from the earth.

▸ Make eye contact: Look for a friendly face in the audience (perhaps someone who is smiling) and make eye contact with them for four or five seconds. Then find someone else to do this with. Making eye contact helps you connect with your listeners and keeps your eyes from darting around nervously.

▸ Admit that you are nervous: Confessing your nervousness to your audience can diminish its power and help you relax. Say it with humor, if you like, but be sure to practice any jokes before your speech.

▸ Have a ready referral: Have a list of other sources on your subject. If someone asks a question that you cannot answer, refer them to what they might read or who they might talk to rather than trying to bluff your way through the answer.

▸ Relativize: Remember, this is just a talk, not a matter of life or death. Don't let your fear convince you otherwise.

4
Anger

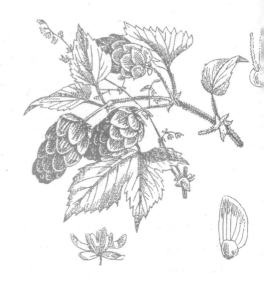

Circumstance does not make the man; it reveals him to himself.

JAMES ALLEN, *As a Man Thinketh*

Anger is a common emotion in everyday life. We can become angry when our desire for something or someone meets resistance, or when we don't get what we want, whether it is love, happiness, recognition, reward, justice, money, ease, fame, or respect. We more easily become angry when we are tired, hungry, anxious, or scared.

Anger is also a normal part of the grieving process (see chapter 17) and recovery from trauma (see chapter 18).

It may also be a hormonal problem. Studies show that people who are overly disruptive and behave aggressively often have low levels of serotonin, the feel-good hormone that helps transmit nerve impulses from one neuron to another. Exposure to heavy metals, such as lead, can cause hormonal conditions that contribute to delinquent and angry behavior.

Anger can be beneficial as a driver of change. For example, anger arising from injustice and inequity has driven many civil rights movements. But it's important to differentiate between anger as a motivator and anger as a problem.

Natural remedies can lessen the intensity and frequency of anger by calming the nervous system and helping clear pent up emotions.

Anger
The Traditional Chinese Medicine Perspective

In traditional Chinese medicine, the emotions of anger and depression correlate to the liver. This organ is also said to correspond to the element of Wood, to be enhanced by creativity, and to govern the nervous system, which houses the soul.

An unhealthy liver may aggravate anger, and excessive anger can injure the liver. (Interestingly, the English word *bilious* refers to both bad temper as well as liver problems.) Anger is seen as a hot emotion of ascending chi or liver yang rising. Sudden brutal anger injures the yin and fluids of the body.

Anger is the liver fire rising—stagnant energy has no where to go so it rises up and explodes outward in bursts of anger. To clear anger, the goal in Chinese medicine is to correct the cause, reduce heat, and move stagnation.

Anger in the Body

Anger has an extreme physiological effect. It causes imbalanced respiration (shallow inhalation and strong, panting exhalation), high blood pressure, increased circulation, elevated cholesterol levels, muscle tightness, clenched jaw, and increased stomach (hydrochloric) acid production. It's accompanied by a flood of hormones—catecholamine, adrenaline, noradrenaline—that rev you up for immediate action.

Chronic anger and/or pent-up angry feelings can cause physiological harm, from headaches and high blood pressure to high cholesterol, ulcers, hemorrhoids, cancer, rheumatoid arthritis, and heart disease—not to mention the damage it can do to your psyche and relationships.

Nutritional Therapy

Nutritional therapy focuses on foods that benefit the liver and mellow the emotion of anger. These include artichokes, barley, daikon radishes, green leafy vegetables (especially dandelion greens), lemons, lentils, mung beans, rye, sour green apples, and white beans. Eating foods like nuts can boost serotonin levels.

Skip This!

According to traditional Chinese medicine excessive amounts of garlic, onions, and coffee can be too hot and aggravate anger, making you more likely to fly off the handle.

Supplements for Well-Being

For someone with chronic anger issues, supplements that calm the nervous system and support the liver can be helpful. B-complex vitamins are a good place to start. Another good option is 5-HTP (5-hydroxytryptophan), which can help correct a neurotransmitter imbalance. An amino acid formula containing alanine, arginine, glutamine, histidine, isoleucine, leucine, lysine, methionine, phenylalanine, threonine, and valine can help ease anger, as can a calcium-magnesium supplement. GTF chromium will help balance blood sugar levels, which can contribute to angry feelings. The DHA and EPA in fish oil can also help nourish the brain and promote clear thinking. A tryptophan supplement can boost serotonin levels and calm anger.

Healing Herbs

Herbs that help cool the liver will soothe anger. They include:

Blessed thistle	Oatstraw
Bupleurum	Passionflower
Dandelion root	Peony Root
Dong quai	Skullcap
Licorice root	

Homeopathy

Homeopathic remedies that can cool fire in the liver include:

Chamomilla	Nux vomica
Lachesis	Sepia
Lycopodium	Staphysagria
Mercuris	Sulfur
Natrum muriaticum	

Flower Essences

Flower essences that assist in calming anger include:

- **Cherry Plum:** For those who feel like they are about to do something desperate. For those prone to temper tantrums.

- **Heather:** For those who are easily irritated.

- **Holly:** For jealousy and sibling rivalry.

- **Impatiens:** For those who feel irritable and impatient.

- **Walnut:** To protect against outside influences that cause anger. For those who are going through big life changes.

Aromatherapy

Calming essential oils can be helpful for relieving angry feelings. Use them in a diffuser, inhale five to ten times from the bottle, or use them in a nice, warm bath. Soak your anger away! Good choices include the following:

Basil	Lemon balm
Cardamom	Lotus
Chamomile	Marjoram
Coriander	Neroli
Frankincense	Patchouli

Geranium	Pine
Hyssop	Rose
Jasmine	Ylang-ylang
Lavender	

Mind-Body Therapies and Practices

Bodywork, like massage, can help soften the liver and soothe a savage spirit. Yoga helps by improving flexibility in body and mind. A calming folk remedy is to get buried in the sand, with your face uncovered, of course! Just getting outdoors can boost serotonin levels, making you feel better and more balanced.

Anger is an emotion and is neither good nor bad. What matters is what we do with it. Harming yourself, others, or any living being is wrong and destructive. Finding effective ways to experience, process, and discharge anger, such as the practices listed here, can be positive and healing.

Relax

- As soon as you begin to feel angry, focus on breathing deeply. Affirm that you are angry, rather than being in denial.
- Try counting to ten while visualizing the calming color blue. There may be some occasions where you need to count to one hundred!
- Drink some cold water.

Release

- Try sitting by a train track and screaming as the train rushes by.
- Try punching a pillow, using a punching bag, or using a foam bat to beat up tough furniture.
- Use your anger to get creative. One of my teachers, Michael

Tierra, would say, "Art is toxic discharge." So get out there and paint, write, create music, or find some way to express yourself and contribute to your own therapy.

Communicate

▶ Be clear about what is really bothering you.

▶ If you are having an argument, make eye contact with the person you are arguing with. Listen to what they have to say without interrupting, and do your best to see things from their point of view. Nod or say "yes" to indicate you are listening. Mirror back what they say. Be willing to forgive!

▶ Consider humor a more valuable ally than profanity.

▶ If necessary, remove yourself from a hot situation and return when you can more safely express yourself.

▶ Write an angry letter, but review it when you're feeling calm before you email or mail it. Otherwise, you may come to regret what you've said. Clear, respectful language works best. Without attacking, let your feelings be known.

▶ Write a letter you never intend to send to release angry feelings. Let it ALL out. Get everything off your chest. Vent venomously on paper. Cry and feel your feelings, write your anger, frustrations, confusion. Let writing be a cleanse. Be totally honest.

▶ Perhaps seek a therapist, someone outside the situation, to communicate your emotions to. (Always seek professional council if anger results in harm to yourself or others or thoughts of destructive actions.)

What Not to Do in an Argument

▶ Do not overuse profanity or scream at the other person. It can impair your ability to be heard.

▶ Do not use statements such as "you always" or "you never." Stick with the issue at hand.

▶ Do not resort to name-calling and blaming, going for the jugular, and verbal threats.

▶ Do not use hostile body language (pointing your finger, baring your teeth, and so on) or physical threats (getting really close, pushing, making a fist, and so on). It can aggravate emotions and resolves nothing.

▶ Do not point your finger or use defensive body language, like crossing your arms in front of you.

All of these things can be provocative, potentially escalating the situation or even putting you in danger of physical defense/retaliation.

Write It Down

To put things into perspective, write down and rate the things that make you angry, on a scale from one to ten, with ten being the highest. You may find that some of them are not as important as you thought they were!

Make a list about what aspects of the anger you are accountable for. Write about what you can do to address those aspects. If you are able to express your feelings on paper, you may find yourself in better emotional health overall and more easily able to make amends and be kind to yourself and others.

5
Low Mood
and Depression

Have patience with all things, but chiefly have patience with yourself. Do not lose courage in considering your own imperfections but instantly set about remedying them— every day begin the task anew.

SAINT FRANCIS DE SALES

Depression is more than having an occasional "off day" when things just aren't going your way. It's a pervasive mood that ranges from a mild case of the blues to a dark cloud that follows you around. Depression can affect every aspect of your life, from the way you feel to the thoughts you think, how you sleep, what you eat, and how you interact with others.

Since depression harms the vital energy of the body, it can translate into physical symptoms such as paleness, slumped shoulders, sunken chest, weak arms, and a head that juts forward, as if reflecting a feeling of heaviness and overburden.

Many of us have experienced bouts of depression as a reaction to a traumatic event such as loss of a loved one, an accident, or unwanted changes. You may also suffer from malaise if you're stuck, figuratively speaking, and don't know how to move forward. However, this type of depression is considered a normal reaction and exogenous, meaning due to external factors. Depression becomes a problem when it is severe, chronic, or endogenous, meaning due to internal factors.

Natural remedies can help nourish and correct underlying contributors to depression. They can provide the raw material to help neurotransmitter production and strengthen organs such as the liver and thyroid, which when out of balance can contribute to depression. Remember: These remedies are not a substitute for care from your doctor or therapist if you are moderately to severely depressed. Talk to your doctor about what is right for you.

Why Are You Depressed?

If you can't pinpoint the cause of your depression, it may be due to a biochemical imbalance. For example, low levels of key amino acids such as phenylalanine, tyrosine, and the neurotransmitter dopamine can cause depression. That's because these amino acids are precursors to mood-regulating neurotransmitters called monoamines, such as serotonin, melatonin, norepinephrine, and dopamine. Monoamine oxidase is an enzyme that helps remove the neurotransmitters dopamine, serotonin, and norepinephrine from the brain.

Monoamine oxidase inibitors (MAOIs) are one type of antidepressant drug used to prevent the removal of these mood-blancing neurotransmitters. Another common antidepressant drug type are selective serotonin reuptake inhibitors (SSRIs). These drugs focus on increasing serotonin levels. While drug treatments can be effective and even life-saving at times, they often cover up the cause.

Natural remedies can help us correct the cause. It's important to find out why a depressed person's serotonin is low—protein deficient? EPA deficient? However, if a person is on medication, they should always speak with their doctor or a competent health care professional before getting off or decreasing their medications or adding in natural supplements. Some combinations of medications can be potentiated by using herbs or supplements that have a similar effect and one ends up with a double dose!

Depression runs in families, so if your parent suffers from this condition, you may too. Other factors include hypothyroidism, which means your body isn't producing enough thyroid hormone, and conditions like chronic fatigue, fibromyalgia, and Lyme disease.

Certain drugs can make you more prone to depression, such as progesterone, estrogen, cortisone, barbiturates, amphetamines, and L-dopa. Depression can be aggravated by food sensitivities and allergies that cause cerebral inflammation. Depressed people often have digestive disorders, including constipation and inflammation.

Good to Know!

In traditional Chinese medicine, depression is said to result from a stagnant condition of the liver. Anger is said to be the result of liver energy rising, and depression is more of an inward movement, where anger is turned against oneself. How does the liver get stagnant? Stuffing down emotions without expressing them doesn't help, and neither does keeping things inside.

Symptoms of Depression

Below are a list of symptoms from the Mayo Clinic website. They note that during a depressive episode symptoms occur most of the day, nearly every day.

- ► Feelings of sadness, tearfulness, emptiness, or hopelessness
- ► Angry outbursts, irritability or frustration, even over small matters
- ► Loss of interest or pleasure in most or all normal activities, such as sex, hobbies, or sports
- ► Sleep disturbances, including insomnia or sleeping too much
- ► Tiredness and lack of energy, so even small tasks take extra effort

- Reduced appetite and weight loss or increased cravings for food and weight gain
- Anxiety, agitation, or restlessness
- Slowed thinking, speaking, or body movements
- Feelings of worthlessness or guilt, fixating on past failures, or self-blame
- Trouble thinking, concentrating, making decisions, and remembering things
- Frequent or recurrent thoughts of death, suicidal thoughts, suicide attempts, or suicide
- Unexplained physical problems, such as back pain or headaches

Keep in mind that these symptoms can indicate other disorders or health conditions, so if you think you or a loved one might be depressed, ask your health care practitioner for help in making a diagnosis. If you are feeling seriously depressed, even suicidal, see your doctor immediately or go to your local emergency room.

If you're feeling blue or have been diagnosed with depression, ask for the help of friends and family members. You don't need to go through this alone.

For those who have mild to moderate depression, the following nutritional and holistic therapies can begin to help put your life back into balance. In fact, Harvard researchers found that more than half of people who have depression and anxiety use alternative medicine to get well.

Nutritional Therapy

Since nutrition affects the structure and function of the brain, it makes sense that healing depression means eating differently. Focus on the following.

The best diet for depression is to consume small, frequent meals with plenty of complex carbohydrates to keep blood sugar levels at an even keel. Complex carbs like amaranth, barley, black rice, brown rice, buckwheat, millet, oatmeal, quinoa, spelt, and teff are digested more slowly, which keeps you off the blood sugar roller coaster. They also increase levels of serotonin, the happy hormone, in your brain. Oatmeal, in particular, also possesses many healthful antioxidant and anti-inflammatory compounds, including carotenoids, tocotrienols (vitamin E), flavonoids, and polyphenols.

Skip This!

Avoid hydrogenated or partially hydrogenated oils hidden in bread, cookies, crackers, and chips. Poor quality oils congest the liver, making it work overtime. Poor liver function can be a large factor in depression according to the principles of traditional Chinese medicine. Sweets and simple carbs like white rice and bread give you a quick boost but also spike insulin levels, which then lead to a drop in blood sugar; you may even feel worse than you did earlier.

Beans, nuts, seeds, tempeh, tofu, fish, meat, eggs, and dairy (of course from high-quality organic sources) all provide protein, which helps keep blood sugar stable, and are rich in B vitamins that balance your mood by improving neurotransmitter function. According to a 2010 study in the *American Journal of Clinical Nutrition,* older adults who are deficient in B vitamins have a higher risk of depression. Nuts and seeds like cashews, almonds, sunflower seeds, and pumpkin seeds are also all high in magnesium, which helps the body produce more serotonin and improves energy. Two ripe bananas a day are also said to help the production of serotonin and norepinephrine. In addition to its benefit as a protein, fish also contains omega-3 fatty acids, which help neurons function optimally and increase gray matter, so we can focus and think clearly and also stabilize mood. Eat cold-water fish like cod, wild salmon, herring, and mackerel three times a week to fill up on omega fatty acids or supplement with a high-quality fish oil high in eicosapentaenoic acid (EPA).

Good to Know!

Foods that are sour and bitter help move liver stagnation. Adding the juice of half a lemon to a glass of water helps stimulate the flow of bile and improves digestion.

Supplements for Well-Being

Not getting enough B-complex vitamins can lead to irritability and mental sluggishness. Folic acid also influences your mood. Low levels of folic acid can also determine whether or not talk therapy or prescription drug therapy is useful. This nutrient even improves how well antidepressants work and helps minimize their side effects.

Calcium and magnesium are essential for nerve and muscle function. Look for chelate or citrate calcium.

SAM-e (S-adenosyl-L-methionine) is an amino acid found in every cell, with the highest concentrations in the brain, adrenal glands, and liver. It helps relieve depression by raising levels of the neurotransmitters serotonin and dopamine and making the receptors for these compounds more available. It also increases levels of melatonin, aids in the production of glutathione, and improves energy. SAM-e breaks down into homocysteine, which is inflammatory, so be sure to get adequate B vitamins to reduce homocysteine levels if you are taking SAM-e as a supplement.

DL-phenylalanine (DLPA) works to heal depression in two ways: It stimulates endorphin, norepinephrine, and noradrenaline production, and it inhibits the enzymes that break down the body's natural feel-good endorphins, so that they survive longer. It works best for depression coupled with low energy, a sense of helplessness, and low self-esteem. It can also help if your blues are the result of change, like the loss of a loved one. It has also been found to ameliorate the depressive phases of bipolar disorder, schizophrenia, premenstrual syndrome, and drug withdrawal.

Mother Nature's News

Research shows that both oral and intravenous SAM-e are of value in the treatment of mild to moderate depression. A 2002 review by the U.S. Agency for Healthcare Research and Quality revealed that SAM-e was more effective than placebo at relieving depression.

L-tyrosine, a precursor for the happy hormone serotonin, can be helpful for those with too little noradrenaline or dopamine activity. Try taking it in the morning and midafternoon. Tryptophan, an amino acid that helps the body produce serotonin, can help lift depression and is another supplement to consider.

Healing Herbs

Herbs can offer a safe and healthful alternative to prescription medications without side effects. However, if you are taking medication, do not stop taking it without getting your doctor's approval. Not all herbs are appropriate for everyone (such as during pregnancy, with high blood pressure, etc.), so seeking out a competent healthcare professional can be important. Also seek your doctor's approval before you begin taking herbal remedies in conjunction with your medication; using both at the same time may have unpredictable results.

Some herbs that can help improve depression follow.

- **Dandelion root:** Improves liver function by stimulating bile production.

🍃 **Eleuthero:** Helps you better cope with stress and relieves depression, fatigue, and insomnia.

🍃 **Ginkgo:** Improves circulation and helps the brain utilize oxygen better, which can help elevate mood and memory. Increases cellular glucose uptake and improves neural transmission. Helps preserve omega-3 fatty acid levels to improve mood.

🍃 **Goji berries:** Traditionally used to promote cheerfulness.

🍃 **Kava kava:** Good for mild depression and anxiety.

🍃 **Lavender:** Its uplifting aroma helps alleviate fear, anxiety, exhaustion, and depression.

🍃 **Lemon balm:** Traditionally used to relieve melancholy, depression, and anxiety. Can help you cope with difficult life situations. The famous Arabian physician Avicenna said of this herb, "It causeth the mind and heart to be merry." It acts upon the autonomic nervous system, protecting the brain from excessive external stimuli.

🍃 **Licorice root:** Helps keep blood sugar levels stable.

🍃 **Motherwort:** Traditionally used for anxiety, depression, exhaustion, gloom, and overworry.

🍃 **Oatstraw:** Rich in nerve-nourishing nutrients. It aids convalescence, debility, drug addiction, exhaustion, insomnia, and post-traumatic stress.

🍃 **Rhodiola:** Improves mild to moderate depression.

🍃 **Yerba maté:** Brightens the mood and provides a plethora of minerals that nourish every aspect of the body (it does contain some caffeine, so is more appropriate for morning use, as it can be energizing).

Saint John's wort is perhaps the best-known herbal remedy for depression and low mood. It acts in a similar way to selective serotonin reuptake inhibitor (SSRI) antidepressant drugs, such as Prozac. Research suggests that a Saint John's wort supplement taken once a day may be as effective as the prescription drug sertraline (Zoloft) for people with mild to moderate depression. This herb inhibits both MAO-A and MAO-B, slowing down the breakdown of neurotransmitters norepinephrine and serotonin, and is rich in flavonoids and amino acids such as glutamine and lysine. Unlike prescription medications, it doesn't have side effects such as dry mouth, nausea, headache, or sexual dysfunction.

!

Cure Caution

If you are already taking antidepressants, talk to your doctor before taking Saint John's wort. This herb can affect and interact with other prescription medications, like birth control pills, drugs used to control HIV infection, anticancer drugs, and drugs that help prevent organ rejection. It can also make you more sensitive to sunlight.

Chinese Patent Medicine

Xiao Yao Wan, also known as Bupleurum Sedative Pills or Free and Easy Pills, is an herbal formula from traditional Chinese medicine that encourages the free-flowing energy of the liver, thus relieving stagnation and improving circulation, easing stress, calming irritability, and improving depression. Da Chai Hu Wan or Great Bupleurum Pills are specific for those with severe depression and a tendency to constipation. You can find these pills in natural health food stores and online.

Homeopathy

Below is a list of homeopathic remedies that can be used to relieve depression in specific types of personalities.

- **Arsenicum album:** Use if you tend to be suspicious and demanding or dislike being in a situation over which you have no control.

Aurum metallicum: Use for depression resulting from personal trauma when you feel in despair and worthless. A classic remedy for suicidal thoughts.

Capsicum: For those who dwell in the past, feel homesick and irritable, or want to be somewhere else.

Causticum: For those depressed due to death of a parent or friend.

Gelsemium: For those with mild depression following illness such as the flu.

Ignatia: Use for disappointment in love or death.

Lachesis: For those whose depression is worse in the morning and during transitions such as menopause and from loss of love. The person may be very talkative and speak without listening.

Natrum muriaticum: For those whose depression is due to disappointment, tragedy, rejection, or betrayal.

Natrum sulphuricum: For those with depression following a head injury.

Pulsatilla: Use if depression alternates with a mild, easygoing manner.

Sepia: Use for emotional issues due to homronal imbalance, such as postpartum blues and mestrual-related depression.

Silicea: Use for melancholy with difficulty concentrating.

Good to Know!
Postpartum Depression

Postpartum depression affects many women in the first year or so after birth and most women experience some form of the "baby blues" in the immediate postpartum period. Natural remedies to support balance during this time include DHA, blessed thistle tea, and Saint John's wort as capsules or a tincture. Homeopathic remedies to consider include sepia, good for those who are experiencing weepiness, exhaustion, and indifference, and ignatia, good for those experiencing postpartum depression accompanied by hysteria and disappointment. Don't hesitate to seek help and advice from a trusted health care practitioner.

Flower Essences

Bach Flower Remedies can help heal emotional imbalances like a blue mood or mild depression. They are very gentle and can safely be taken in combination with medications for depression. Try the following.

- **Agrimony:** For those who hide their depression with a cheerful façade as well as with drugs and alcohol.

- **Crab Apple:** For feelings of uncleanness.

- **Gentian:** Helps with discouragement from setbacks, hopelessness, or despair; for those who are easily discouraged.

- **Gorse:** For hopelessness, despair, despondency, or feelings of inevitable trouble.

- **Hornbeam:** For when you're blue, gloomy, or mentally fatigued.

- **Mustard:** For depression that comes and goes suddenly, with no known cause.

- **Star of Bethlehem:** For trauma, grief, and loss.

- **Sweet Chestnut:** For anguish, bereavement, hopelessness, and despair. For when you feel like you have reached the limits of your endurance.

Aromatherapy

Simply taking deep breaths can help brighten moods as getting more oxygen to the brain can stimulate and open neural pathways. Adding essential oils can help lift your spirits even more. Below is a list of essential oils that are traditionally used for depression, but the most important thing is that you enjoy the smell of the oil. Having an assortment of oils handy—such as by your desk or in your backpack or purse—can alter the direction a mood is going in a matter of seconds.

Basil	Orange
Bergamot	Palmarosa
Cedarwood	Patchouli
Chamomile	Peppermint
Cinnamon	Rose
Clary sage	Rose geranium
Clove	Rosemary
Coriander	Rosewood
Geranium	Sandalwood
Grapefruit	Spruce
Lavender	Tangerine
Lemon balm	Thyme
Jasmine	Vetiver
Marjoram	Ylang-ylang
Neroli	Wintergreen

To utilize the benefits of these oils you could simply take five deep inhalations on each nostril several times a day. Put the essential oils in a diffuser and fill your bedroom or office with a soothing scent. Put a few drops on your pillow so you inhale the scent as you go to sleep. Shower with an aromatherapy soap. If you're feeling brave, end your shower with cold water to help you feel alive and invigorated!

Mind-Body Therapies and Practices

Natural remedies are not only about what we put in and on our bodies, but also the lifestyle choices we make throughout each day. Find a few lifestyle techniques that you enjoy and do your best to engage in at least a couple each day, perhaps using different techniques on different days. Additionally, hands-on therapies like massage and acupressure can do wonders in alleviating a blue mood or mild depression.

Mother Nature's News

Acupuncture is a promising treatment for depression in women, who are more prone to this condition. University of Arizona researchers studied thirty-eight women with mild to moderate depression and found that, after twelve sessions, 70 percent of the women experienced at least a 50 percent reduction in symptoms, which is comparable to the success rate of psychotherapy and medication.

Researchers at Boston University School of Medicine and McLean Hospital found that practicing yoga increased GABA (gamma-aminobutyric acid) levels, which can help ease depression. The effect was similar to that of treatment with antidepressants. Yoga poses to relieve depression include Cobra, Camel, headstand, and shoulder stand.

Acupressure

Try these acupressure points either as part of a massage or by themselves. Just apply pressure three times for ten seconds each (unless otherwise noted), several times daily.

- ▶ Press the point 1½ inches below the navel.
- ▶ Press right below and on the inside corner of the fingernail of the middle finger.

▶ Press directly below the inside corner of the nail of the pinkie finger.

▶ Place four fingers into the hollow at the base of the skull. Pushing firmly, massage slowly in a circular motion for three minutes.

▶ Apply pressure between the first, second, and third thoracic vertebrae all at once.

Massage

Getting a massage once a week is more than a luxury; it improves circulation and removes blockages in the body. Try a whole-body massage, preferably using one of the essential oils mentioned on page 70 diluted in a carrier oil. If you're feeling blue, ask the practitioner to pay special attention to the back of the neck, the ears, face, chest, shoulders, legs, and feet.

Exercise

Exercise boosts your intake of oxygen, wakes up the body, and stimulates endorphin production, which can mean a more alert, happier, calmer you.

Mother Nature's News

Researchers at the University of Toronto found that moderate exercise can even prevent depression from occurring. The study published in the *American Journal of Preventive Medicine* in 2013 reviewed more than twenty-six years of research findings and discovered that even low levels of physical activity such as walking and gardening for twenty to thirty minutes a day can ward off depression in all age groups.

Go Outside

Spending time in the beauty of nature can be inspiring, whether it be a forest, a beach, or a spectacular mountaintop, and is an excellent way to improve your mood. It also will reduce stress, boost energy, improve sleep, lower blood pressure, enhance immunity, and improve your ability to focus. Brigitte finds that sitting by a river is a reminder to let go of negative emotions and go with the flow.

Keep Your Hands Busy

Art and creating with your hands can be an opportunity for self expression. It doesn't need to be perfect, sellable, or even beautiful. According to the principles of traditional Chinese medicine, creativity helps alleviate anger and depression. Sew, knit, work with wood, sketch, garden, paint. Not only can it help alleviate depression, but it can bolster self-esteem and be a form of active meditation.

Good to Know
Seasonal Affective Disorder (SAD)

In the winter, when days get shorter, the reduction in sunlight can lead to depression and fatigue. These natural therapies can help:

- Get outdoors in full-spectrum light for at least a few minutes a day, preferably without glasses, sunglasses, or even contacts.
- Spend time indoors under a full-spectrum light. A full-spectrum bulb will give you a good dose of sunshine-like light to stimulate your pineal gland and boost your body's production of serotonin, melatonin, and vitamin D.
- Winter months are when serotonin levels are lowest. Try taking tryptophan as a supplement. It helps your body make serotonin, the feel-good hormone.
- Take vitamin D. The sun helps the body make vitamin D, but in the winter, you may need a supplement.

- Take a brisk walk in the early morning or late afternoon. This can help normalize your body's circadian rhythms, which affect appetite, sleep, temperature, blood pressure, and many other factors in physical and mental health.

- Use a sunrise alarm clock, which slowly brightens as you near your wake-up time.

- Keep your blood sugar stable by eating a healthy diet with plenty of protein, complex carbohydrates, and whole grains and nuts (which also contain vitamins B_6 and B_{12}, which are important for brain health).

Write It Down

It's time to put pen to paper or fingers to the keyboard. Writing about the way you feel can change your perspective and make you feel better.

Write down all the factors that you think might be contributing to your blue mood: losses, difficulties, obstacles. Make a list. See if you can find a way to look at these issues from a more open perspective—as learning experiences, opportunities for change or rebirth, initiators of personal growth. Write those thoughts down too. Return to this list often—review it, update it, keep track of the ways in which your efforts to hold a different perspective affect your mood.

Choose ten activities to accomplish every day, even if they are as simple as getting dressed and making the bed. At night, write down what you did each day that was productive and how it made you feel. Celebrate the positive actions you took. Gradually, this will boost your self esteem and motivate you to continue. Most of all, be kind to yourself along the way.

!

Cure Caution

Natural remedies and lifestyle changes are not a substitute for proper evaluation and mental health care. If depression is not adequately treated, it can become severe and, in some cases, dangerous. Consult a mental health professional if you or someone you care about may be experiencing depression.

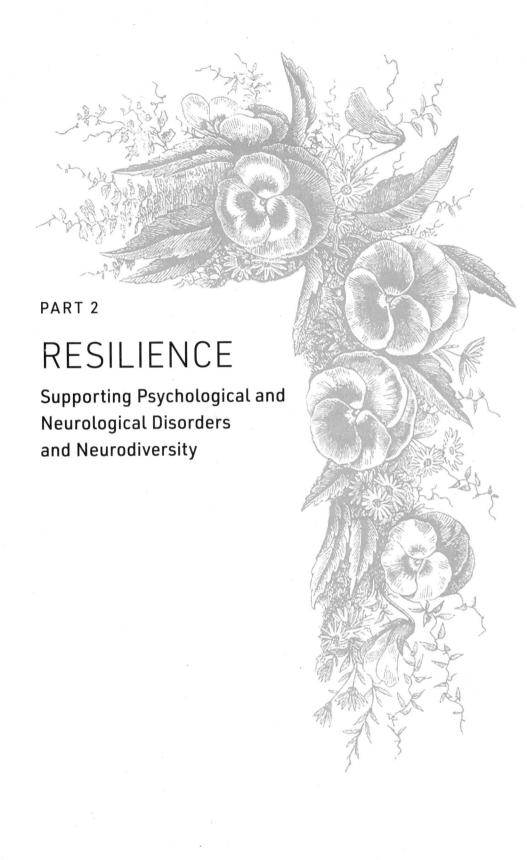

PART 2

RESILIENCE

Supporting Psychological and
Neurological Disorders
and Neurodiversity

!

Caution

The chapters in part 2 focus on serious psychological and neurological disorders that require complex medical treatment. Therefore, the natural remedies offered here should be used as an adjunct treatment within the overall wellness plan from your health care practitioner. Depending on your condition, symptoms may not completely resolve, but many have experienced improvement through the use of these natural modalities. The remedies given here are meant to provide you and your health care practitioner as many tools as possible to improve your overall wellness.

6
Addiction

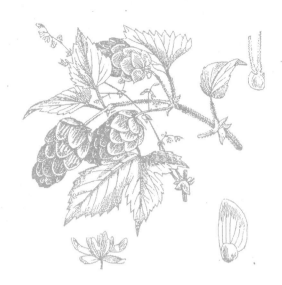

Genetic, environmental, and developmental factors, on their own or in combination, play an influential role in determining the risk for addiction. Addiction itself can bring on psychological and emotional problems, or it can be the result of them. Treatment options vary widely, depending on the addiction and the person. Twelve-step support groups can be a big help, as can counseling or therapy, and working with your doctor and other trained mental health professionals.

Natural remedies for addiction focus on easing the emotional and mental health issues that can arise with addiction and withdrawal, as well as reducing cravings, supporting the nervous system, cleansing the liver, and rebuilding overall health. Natural remedies can nourish, calm, improve brain chemistry imbalances, and increase energy levels, all of which can help us to get through challenging times in life instead of choosing self destructive behaviors. (For more extensive information on natural remedies for addiction, check out Brigitte's book *Addiction-Free Naturally*.)

Nutritional Therapy

When recovering from addiction, focus on cleansing, rebuilding, and nurturing yourself. Focus on foods that help the liver cleanse itself, such as apples, artichokes, beets, burdock root, carrots, celery, daikon radish, green leafy vegetables, persimmons, and hemp seed oil. Drink the juice of half a lemon in water several times daily to help detoxify the liver.

Good to Know!

There may be a correlation between addiction and blood sugar problems. It may be wise to cut back on or give up sugar and other simple carbohydrates, such as processed flour products, if you have addictive tendencies. Check out *Beat Sugar Addiction Now!* by Jacob Teitelbaum, M.D. and Chrystle Fiedler for more information.

Look to sea vegetables to help nourish the thyroid gland and endocrine system, which may have become damaged by the use of deleterious substances. Superfoods like blue-green algae, spirulina, and chlorella can be highly nutritive and rebuilding.

Supplements for Well-Being

Vitamin C is detoxifying and can reduce cravings. A calcium-magnesium supplement is especially helpful in giving the nervous system support and promoting calmness. B-complex vitamins help diminish withdrawal symptoms and aid liver regeneration. A supplement of GTF chromium helps the body regulate blood sugar levels and metabolize carbohydrates.

Healing Herbs

Herbs that can help you overcome addiction include the following.

- 🍃 **Basil:** A nerve restorative that lifts the spirits from depression and calms anxiety.

- 🍃 **Cinnamon:** Improves circulation and is stimulating yet calming to the nerves. Cinnamon is naturally sweet, thereby satisfying the body's desires for other substances.

🍃 **Clove:** Helps reduce cravings and is a natural antioxidant, expectorant, and stimulant.

🍃 **Dandelion root:** Helps detoxify the body, cleansing the liver and stimulating digestion.

🍃 **Fennel seed:** Naturally sweet, which helps stabilize blood sugar levels and thereby decreases the desire for substances while improving energy levels.

🍃 **Lemon balm:** Helps during withdrawal and detox periods by lifting the spirits and supporting the nervous system.

🍃 **Milk thistle seed:** Can be used to help rebuild a damaged liver.

🍃 **Oatstraw:** Calms and strengthens the nerves, lessens anxiety, and decreases the desire for substances.

🍃 **Saint John's wort:** Can help relieve the depression and anxiety that causes you to turn to addictive substances for temporary relief.

🍃 **Skullcap:** Calms the emotions, enhances awareness, and quiets overexcitability. It helps curb the emotional need and cravings for addictive substances.

Note: Anyone suffering from alcoholism should use herbs in the form of teas, glycerites, or capsules rather than as tinctures, which contain alcohol.

Aromatherapy

Essential oils can be most helpful in giving up an addiction. Every time you crave an addictive substance, take deep inhalations of essential oils such as basil cardamom, fennel, and/or rosemary. These oils fill some of the same receptor sites as abused substances and can provide immediate sensory pleasure to the brain—without harm—as the nasal passages are in such close proximity. You can also try them in a bath; add one pound of Epsom salts and eight to ten drops of any of these essential oils to the warm water, then get in and soak to relax and detox your system.

Mind-Body Therapies and Practices

Taking action to find support mentally and physically, change habits, and rethink the way you look at the world all serve to advance recovery and promote well-being. Addiction keeps us stuck and impairs our ability to grow. So stop postponing—this is the moment! You deserve to be happy and free. The first step is to admit there is a problem. The second step is to do something about it. Consider these holistic wellness suggestions; try the ones that speak to you and see what happens!

Good to Know!

Consider psychedelic therapy—with a trained guide. Psychedelics are again being studied and shown to help in treatment of depression, cluster headaches, OCD, post traumatic stress, anxiety, alcoholism, and addiction.

Acupuncture

Acupuncture has helped many people overcome addiction because of its ability to stimulate detoxification.

Practical Tips for Recovery from Addiction

Find support. Ask friends and family members for help. Find a twelve-step program for support and connection. Recovery can be a long and difficult path. That's why it's important to connect with others on the same road. Members of 12 step groups such as AA and NA offer experience, strength, and hope while making you feel less alone and more empowered.

Learn from experience. Ask other people who have given up an addiction how they did it and how their success has benefited them.

Substitute. Replace a negative behavior with a positive one. For example, instead of having coffee every morning, go for a walk. Instead of having a drink every night, take an aromatherapy bath or call a friend.

Tackle something new. Take up a new activity or a craft. Learning something new distracts the mind, keeps you busy, and can help improve your self-esteem.

List your reasons. Make a list of the reasons why you should give up an addiction. Put it where you can often read it—above a sink, on a mirror, on a bookmark, in your wallet. Being clear about why you want to give up an addiction is very important to strengthen your determination in letting go of what no longer serves you and your life.

Visualize. Draw a picture of your addiction to help you gain perspective. For example, you might draw a monkey on your back—the classic metaphor for addiction.

See yourself. Have someone photograph you while you are indulging in your addiction. Look into the camera as they snap your photo. Look carefully at the photo and ask yourself what it is trying to tell you.

Unveil your inner child. Try writing to your addiction with your dominant hand, describing how it affects you. Then, with your non-dominant hand, have your addiction "write back to you" as a way to tap into your sunconscious and help reveal some of your inner child behavior.

Use color as therapy. The color blue helps you relax and cools inflammation. Green is balancing. Wear or surround yourself with these colors when you can.

Breathe! Deep breathing is calming as well as energizing and provides your brain with a much-needed substance: oxygen. Exercise also increases the amount of oxygen available to the body.

Keep track. Be consistent and keep track of your progress, such as posting it on the refrigerator. Consider showing the progress chart to someone you really trust. Tell them you are sharing your progress with them as a method of accountability, not because you want them to nag you. But if there are ways they can help you stay consistent, tell them.

Declutter. Do what it takes to have a clean, uncluttered place so your consciousness will not be encumbered. Keeping a planner, whether on paper or digital, can help your mind feel more organized so that life feels less stressful.

Nurture yourself. Good nutrition, massage, biofeedback, hypnotism, exercise, meditation, and prayer may all be healing on deep levels. Find ways to reward yourself each day—a massage, a foot rub, and a long-distance phone call to a favorite friend . . .

Fulfill your true spiritual quest. What do you believe in? What matters most? Find out and then do something about it!

Stay positive. Learn to deal with any lapses in a positive, healing way. Be a free, conscious being.

Best wishes to all of you who are brave enough to let go of that which does not benefit your life!

7
Eating Disorders

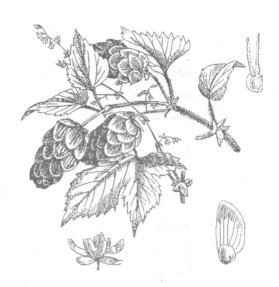

In this section we focus on two of the most common eating disorders, anorexia and bulimia. Natural remedies can be useful tools for both of these conditions to calm stress and anxiety, nourish the body, boost appetite, and improve diegestion.

!
Cure Caution

Both anorexia and bulimia are serious conditions and can be life threatening, so it's important to work with a trusted health care practitioner to help you get well. The information you'll read here is meant as a complement to, not a substitute for, professional health care. Check with your health care practitioner to see whether these natural remedies might be right for you.

Anorexia and bulimia are much more likely to occur in women than men; about 90 percent of cases are female. Anorexia is chronic undereating, driven by distorted body image and an intense fear of weight gain. It can be diagnosed when weight loss leads to a body weight that is 85 percent or less of what is considered normal.

Anorexia can lead to amenorrhea, anemia, hair loss, constipation, low blood pressure, edema, sleep disturbances, nutritional deficiency, hypothermia, hypoglycemia, hirsutism, osteoporosis later in life, cardiac episodes, and emaciation as well as a lifetime of digestive disorders.

Bulimia is a repeated cycle of bingeing (eating excessively) and then purging, either by vomiting or through the abuse of laxatives. The repeated vomiting, in particular, can have devastating effects upon the teeth, stomach, and esophagus, such as dental erosion, bone loss, and life long digestive disorders.

Anorexia and bulimia are classified as separate psychiatric disorders, but sometimes they overlap. Both conditions result, in part, from having abnormally low levels of endorphins, the feel-good hormones. Fasting, bingeing, purging, excessive dieting, starving oneself, and overexercising all elevate endorphin levels, but only temporarily, which can result in a cycle of negative behavior that is very difficult to change. Both of these conditions also often result, in part, from depression and anxiety and/or lead to these conditions, so many of the natural remedies target these aspects of the disorders. These conditions should be taken seriously—people can die from both of these eating disorders.

These three steps can help you begin to heal from anorexia and/or bulimia:

The Three Steps to Healing

1. Correct any underlying health problem (such as low thyroid function, a biochemical imbalance, or unidentified food allergens).
2. Establish healthy eating patterns and regain weight, if necessary, to bring you out of danger of physical impairment.
3. Get counseling by a professional with expertise in helping people with eating disorders.

There are many natural therapies and practices that can support this work of healing.

Nutritional Therapy

Eating a varied diet that is nutrient dense, easy to digest, and health giving can help you reach a healthy weight if you have an eating disorder. Increase food levels gradually as you heal.

Taking a dose of digestive bitters, which contain herbs like centaury, gentian, and orange peel, ten minutes before a meal can increase appetite and aid digestion.

Skip This

Avoid common allergens, food intolerances, and yeast producers such as gluten, sugar, alcohol, and some dairy products. Intolerance or allergies of certain foods can damage the intestinal lining. This may create discomfort when eating more nourishing but hard to digest foods, which in turn may create a cycle of fear around food that can exacerbate disordered eating. Simlarly yeast overgrowth can cause people to feel bloated when they consume carbohydrates, which can, in turn, lead to anxiety about food and poor body image.

Nourishing foods that are easy to digest, such as blended, soaked, fermented, baked, or sprouted foods, can be an easier way to assimilate in a way that feels safe for those whose digestion may be impaired from an eating disorder.

When you're recovering from an eating disorder, also eliminate caffeine, which can aggravate feelings of anxiety and depression.

According to the principles of traditional Chinese medicine, the earth element governs the stomach and spleen and issues that affect the digestive system, high and low blood sugar, and eating disorders in general. It's also important to focus on foods that calm the spirit, nourish the stomach and spleen, and tonify the heart, like pumpkins, winter squash, and sweet potatoes. Watery black quinoa, millet, or black rice with some cooked vegetables would be ideal as as these nourishing foods in their softer form are easier to digest. Use seasonings such as cilantro, cinnamon, garlic, and ginger, which increase "digestive fire"—improving circulation to the digestive organs and improving assimilation of nutrients. Raw juices, smoothies, soups, and blended foods can combine several foods that are easy to swallow or chew as well as to assimilate into the digestive system. Persimmons and ripe pineapple, both rich in enzymes that aid digestion, are good fruits to include.

Supplements for Well-Being

Both anorexia and bulimia are associated with low levels of zinc, so you may want to supplement with this mineral. Zinc also improves the senses of smell and taste, which can improve appetite. Studies indicate that zinc in a sulfate form is most effective, and a liquid form, which is most absorbable, is ideal, given that eating disorders can cause low hydrochloric acid production in the stomach.

Calcium and magnesium are nourishing to the nervous system and can help prevent further bone loss, leading to likeliness of fractures. Iron in a chelated form can help correct anemia. Essential fatty acids found in a high-quality fish oil and a B-complex vitamin help stabilize the emotional body. Beta-carotene can help heal mucous membranes in the body, which can be irritated from lack of nourishment as well as from vomiting and laxative use in the case of bulimia.

Supplementation with amino acids can also be helpful in recovery. L-glutamine helps stabilize blood sugar and enhances mental clarity. Tryptophan is needed to make serotonin, which helps balance emotions, aids sleep, and controls pain. L-tyrosine can reduce depression and is a precursor to serotonin. D-phenylalanine works as an antidepressant and is used to make adrenaline and tyrosine.

SAM-e can help elevate mood by elevating levels of serotonin, dopamine, and phosphatides. It's needed for neuronal membrane integrity, neurotransmitter synthesis, and energy metabolism. It also increases the binding of neurotransmitters to receptors and improves the fluidity of brain cell membranes, all of which help emotional stability.

Healing Herbs

The following herbs can help ease the symptoms of anorexia and bulimia and encourage appetite. Many of these herbs address physical symptoms, such as various types of discomfort throughout the digestive system, while others address some of the mental and emotional causes and symptoms of eating disorders. You can take them in tea, tincture, or capsule form.

- **California poppy:** Calms the nerves and helps relieve anxiety and stress.

- **Catnip:** Helps relieve amenorrhea, anxiety, flatulence, indigestion, and nausea.

- **Chamomile:** Restores an exhausted nervous system.

- **Cloves:** Used to treat depression, flatulence, indigestion, stomach cramps, and vomiting.

- **Dandelion:** The leaves help relieve anemia.

- **Eleuthero:** Used for debility and convalescence. It helps with depression, fatigue, and nervous breakdown and gives support during stress.

- **Ginger:** Used to treat amenorrhea, cramps, dyspepsia, flatulence, indigestion, and nausea.

🍃 **Hops:** Used to treat anxiety, indigestion, irritable bowel, and restlessness. They can help you put on weight, improve assimilation of food, stimulate digestive secretions, and calm anxiety and nervousness.

🍃 **Lemon balm:** Helps protect the brain from excessive stimuli and calms anxiety. It benefits depression, nausea, and nervousness.

🍃 **Licorice root:** Soothes an irritated digestive tract, even one raw from vomiting. It also improves debility, emotional instability, indigestion, and stress.

🍃 **Marshmallow root:** Soothes an irritated digestive tract, even one raw from vomiting. It is demulcent, nutritive, and calms the nervous system.

🍃 **Oatstraw:** Nutritive and supportive for the nervous system. It is helpful for debility associated with appetite loss, as well as anxiety, convalescence, depression, exhaustion, and stress.

🍃 **Passionflower:** Quiets the central nervous system and is anti-inflammatory, nervine, and sedative. It is helpful for anxiety, anger, hysteria, nervous breakdown, and stress.

🍃 **Peppermint and spearmint:** Improve dyspepsia, fatigue, flatulence, indigestion, irritable bowel, nausea, stomachache, and stress.

🍃 **Saint John's wort:** Inhibits the breakdown of serotonin, while enhancing its efficiency. Use it for anxiety, depression, and irritability.

🍃 **Skullcap:** Enhances awareness and calmness and aids anxiety, emotional trauma, fear, hysteria, and stress.

🍃 **Slippery elm bark:** Soothes an irritated, raw digestive tract, helping to rebuild its mucosal lining.

Chinese Patent Medicine

A Chinese patent formula to consider is Ren Shen Yang Ying Wan, which nourishes the heart and spleen and calms the spirit. Another is Shih Chuan Da Bu Wan (Ten Flavor Tea), which tonifies the heart, spleen, and blood and improves poor appetite and digestion, debility, and anxiety.

Homeopothy

Homeopathic remedies to consider for eating disorders include:

- **Aconitum napellus:** For fright that causes appetite loss.

- **Arsenicum album:** For exhaustion, vomiting, or fear of poisoning that is worse after eating.

- **Cinchona:** For an eating disorder that started with bulimia. For the person who is very sensitive and theorizes a lot.

- **Gelsemium:** For the person who is quiet, weak, dull, apathetic, and not thirsty either from deficiency of nutrients or from deep insecurities, anxiety, and trauma.

- **Ignatia:** For the person who fears getting fat and rejection and is obsessive about weight.

- **Natrum muriaticum:** For the person with dry skin and lips, who is constipated, very self-conscious, fears rejection, has a drive for perfectionism, and fears getting fat.

- **Phosphoricum acidum:** For the person who is apathetic toward themselves and food.

- **Sepia:** For the person who is irritable and indifferent to life, wants to be alone, and is disgusted by food and odors, which cause nausea.

Flower Essences

Flower essences can help one get to the core of some of the emotional contributors to an eating disorder.

- 🌢 **Cerato:** For those who lack confidence in their own decisions.

- 🌢 **Crab Apple:** For those who feel unclean and have a poor self image.

- 🌢 **Larch:** For those who feel inferior and expect to fail.

- 🌢 **Rock Water:** For those who suppress their inner needs and are hard on themselves.

Particularly useful, Clematis flower essence is for people who have an aversion to the physical world, including themselves. They follow a punishing diet even if it has an adverse effect upon their health. This remedy mellows their attitude and helps them to have a more positive relationship with the world.

Mind-Body Therapies and Practices

Practice prayer, meditation, guided visualization, and yoga to enhance serenity and stability in your life. Professional support, nutritional therapy, and the support of family and friends can help you find the road back to health!

8
Schizophrenia and Bipolar Disorder

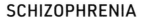

SCHIZOPHRENIA

The term *schizophrenia* derives from the Greek *schizo,* "split," and *phren,* "mind." This disorder is considered one of the most serious mental illnesses, and professional medical care is imperative.

When it comes to natural remedies that can support treatment for schizophrenia, the primary goals are to address nutritional imbalances, relieve stress, and lift depression.

Traditional Chinese medicine considers schizophrenia to be a disorder of excess heat in the heart. The main objective of treatment in this system of healing, then, is to remove phlegm blocking the heart and open the channels of blood circulation.

Nutritional Therapy

Foods to encourage psychological and emotional stability include fish, poultry, peas, sea vegetables, sunflower seeds, and gluten-free whole grains like amaranth, brown rice, and millet. Niacin deficiency is often seen in patients with schizophrenia, so niacin-rich foods like broccoli, carrots, corn, and eggs may be helpful. Focus on eating small, frequent meals to help keep blood sugar levels stable.

Skip This!

As is the case with so many psychological and physical illnesses, food allergies and blood sugar imbalances can be a contributing factor in schizophrenia. Identifying and eliminating food allergens has helped some people with schizophrenia. Also avoid refined grains, which can contribute to hypoglycemia, and nightshade family members (potatoes, eggplants, peppers, tomatoes, tobacco), which can cause inflammation.

Supplements for Well-Being

As noted, many doctors have seen a link between niacin deficiency and schizophrenia. A niacin supplement may be helpful. Note that niacin supplements can sometimes cause a hot, prickly sensation that lasts about ten minutes, though schizophrenics are less prone to niacin flushes.

Interestingly, ingestion of LSD can temporarily mimic the effects of schizophrenia, and niacin is used to gently put a paranoid tripper "back in the driver's seat." Perhaps the same biochemical mechanics are at play?

Niacin is a B vitamin (it's vitamin B_3). Whenever you supplement with a component of the vitamin B complex, it is wise to include the rest of the B complex, separately.

High levels of the neurotransmitter dopamine, which is involved in nerve transmission, can be a factor in schizophrenia. One theory is that many people suffering from schizophrenia are deficient in prostaglandins. Prostaglandins modify the secretion of neurotransmitters like dopamine. Niacin will help in the synthesis of prostaglandins.

Mother Nature's News

Dr. Abram Hoffer, a pioneer in orthomolecular research, studied niacin supplementation in a group of patients with schizophrenia. Seventy-three of the patients took niacin supplements; the other ninety-eight did not. Over the course of three years, seven patients from the niacin group were rehospitalized, compared to forty-seven of those who did not supplement with niacin.

Though it is difficult to acknowledge any benefits of smoking tobacco, nicotine appears to increase circulation to the cerebral cortex and temporarily reduces negative symptoms of schizophrenia. It is sometimes used by patients as an antidepressant and stress reliever and to promote concentration.

Other Supplements to Consider

- **Chromium:** Helps balance blood sugar levels.

- **Evening primrose oil:** High in omega-3 fatty acids, which can reduce nerve and brain inflammation.

- **GABA:** Can sometimes reduce some of the symptoms of schizophrenia by minimizing the brain's response to excitatory messages.

- **Lecithin:** Can help support the nervous system.

- **Melatonin:** Can help improve sleep and decrease schizophrenic episodes as most people with schizophrenia have low nighttime melatonin levels.

- **N-acetylcysteine:** Can help reduce some of the symptoms of schizophrenia.

- **Vitamin E:** Can interfere with anxiety impulses to the brain.

Healing Herbs

Nervines can help lessen symptoms of schizophrenia as they have a calming effect on the nervous system. Good choices include:

Blue vervain	Hyssop
Calamus root	Lavender
Chamomile	Lemon balm
Dandelion root	Saint John's wort
Ginkgo	Skullcap
Gotu kola	Valerian
Hops	Wood betony

Homeopathy

Homeopathic Lithium carbonicum uses the energetics of lithium (in other words an extremely minute dose of lithium that is potentized by the homeopathic process). Therefore one can have the benefits of lithium without the side effects that come with the lithium drug. Of course, one should talk to a competent helth professional before changing or discontinuing a prescription.

!

Cure Caution

When using supplements, herbs, or other natural remedies to help support the treatment of schizophrenia, what works will depend on the individual. If any natural remedy worsens your symptoms, consult with a qualified health care practitioner or try a different remedy.

Aromatherapy

Smelling essential oils can open neural pathways in the brain, producing a calming effect. Essential oils to use for schizophrenia include lavender, lemon balm, orange, and rose geranium.

Mind-Body Therapies and Practices

Daily exercise is most important. Yoga, massage, and chiropractic adjustments can help the body be in alignment so that the necessary chi (or energy/life force) gets to the brain. Gentle breathing (not kundalini) can also be helpful.

BIPOLAR DISORDER

Bipolar disorder (formerly called manic depression) is a biochemical imbalance leading to manic and/or depressive episodes lasting for days. Manic episodes are extreme highs characterized by euphoria, high energy, or high irritability. Depressive episodes are deep lows characterized by sadness, hopelessness, or even suicidal thoughts. Both can affect one's sleep, judgment, behavior, and ability to think clearly. Excessive neurotransmitters, especially norepinephrine, contribute to mania, whereas a deficiency can lead to despair. Fostering a balanced life with regular meals, regular bed times, and grounding on the earth can all be helpful for in keeping the emotional rollercoaster on an even keel.

Lithium is commonly prescribed as a mood-stabilizing treatment for bipolar disorder. It helps smooth out erratic mood cycles, stimulate the reuptake of neurotransmitters and improve the ability of neurotransmitters to communicate with each other. Lithium also appears to help both tryptophan and serotonin circulate longer in the body. Its use dates back to ancient Greece, where lithium-rich sacred mineral springs were used to calm those "gone mad."

Lithium drugs have a *lot* of side effects, including fatigue, upset stomach, nausea, increase in thirst, frequent urination, mental confusion, diarrhea, blurred vision, weight gain, seizures (rare), and a dulling of creativity. Toxic levels of lithium can damage the heart, kidneys and nervous system—and the therapeutic level is very close to the toxic level. Nevertheless, lithium is usually still necessary as part of a treatment protocol.

Some natural alternatives to lithium drugs are explored below. In general, natural remedies can nourish, calm, and support one who might be struggling with the ups and downs of bipolar disorder.

Like schizophrenia, bipolar disorder is a serious mental illness, which can be detrimental to a person's safety and may require drug therapy or hospitalization. A qualified health care provider is essential!

Nutritional Therapy

You can stabilize blood sugar by eating healthy meals at regular intervals—erratic eating can contribute to erratic emotions. Foods and herbs naturally containing lithium include cabbage, coriander, cumin, eggplant, green leafy vegetables, peppers, potatoes, and tomatoes. Lithium also occurs naturally in kelp and oysters. You can also put lemon in water as a good way to get more lithium into the body as the lemon peel contains small amounts of lithium. Though the naturally occurring amounts are smaller, they are more bioavailable, increasing the potency. Consulting with a nutritionally trained health care practitioner is always a good recourse.

Supplements for Well-Being

Supplements that promote mood regulation and help one feel grounded may be one way to help brain chemistry. GABA (gamma-aminobutryic acid) helps induce a sense of calm by inhibiting excitatory messages from reaching the frontal cortex of the brain. A great deal of research has been done on its use in treating bipolar disorder. Studies have shown that the combination of GABA, choline, inositol, and niacinamide are especially sedating, nourishing, and balancing and may be helpful in cases of mania and depression. GABA is especially helpful for manic epidodes, as it calms the brain from being overstimulated by outside influences.

Lithium orotate is available without a prescription and often available at natural food stores. It is thought to have the same benefits as lithium drugs without the same level of side effects. Do consult with a competent health care professional to determine which remedies will be best for you and before stopping any treatments you are currently on.

Other supplements to consider include:

- **B-complex vitamins:** Many people with bipolar disorder are deficient in B vitamins. B vitamins have a calming effect and nourish a nervous system that can be exhausted from being all fired up.

- **Calcium and magnesium:** Taken in a chelated form, these nutrients are helpful in calming the nervous system and can promote stability and groundedness.

- **Tryptophan:** This amino acid can be calming and help in the production of serotonin.

- **Omega-3s:** These essential fatty acids can reduce manic symptoms.

Skip This!

Excessive amounts of sugar, fruit juices, caffeinated beverages, alcohol, and chemical additives like food coloring, preservatives, and even synthetic body care and cleaning products may contribute to the expansive tendency of bipolar mania. Avoid them.

Homeopathy

Some people may find that homeopathic lithium is an effective complement to or supplement for other treatments for mood balance and stability.

Skip This!

Those with bipolar conditions should avoid the amino acids argi-nine and ornithine and the supplement choline as they can be overstimulating. If you are taking MAOIs, avoid tyrosine, which can elevate blood pressure.

Mind-Body Therapies and Practices

Nourishment of the body in many forms can help support the balance of the mind.

Acupressure

Here are a couple of acupressure techniques that can be helpful to calm manic episodes. Just apply pressure three times for ten seconds each (unless otherwise noted).

- ▸ Use the right hand to squeeze the left shoulder muscle to relieve anxiety and tension to stimulate the production of natural opi-ates. Then switch hands.
- ▸ Press one thumbnail into the crease of the wrist on the opposite hand, with the palm facing toward you, and hold for two to three minutes to calm anxiety.
- ▸ Press one thumbnail into the fleshy bulge of the opposite thumb in the center to calm hysteria.

Skip This

Mania can be triggered by Kundalini breath work and, while breath work can be a useful tool, any breathing exercises should be done slowly and cautiously.

Regularity of Schedule

One simple practice that can be beneficial to create balance and stability for those with bipolar disorder is a regular bedtime. As noted, regular mealtimes and regularity of schedule in general can be supportive to other treatments mentioned here.

9
Epilepsy

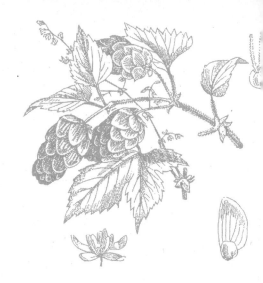

Epilepsy is a disorder characterized by abnormal electrical impulses in the brain, with an adrenaline rush that results in seizures. The seizures, which a patient may or may not remember, can manifest as muscular convulsions, dizziness, frothing at the mouth, headaches, and loss of consciousness. Some people with epilepsy experience pre-seizure prodromes, or premonitory symptoms, including varying sensations, inner voices, music, smells, queasy stomachs, and visual images.

In traditional Chinese medicine, epilepsy is seen as a disorder of the liver. Wind arises from liver deficiency and can contribute to tremors, spasms, and neurological problems. Blockage of the heart meridian by phlegm or dampness or congestion of the system by hot phlegm can also contribute to epilepsy.

Even for those patients for whom seizures occur only infrequently, a healthy lifestyle is key. It may be wise to keep a journal and record your diet, activities, and emotional factors to see if you can find any patterns related to when seizures occur.

Natural remedies and holistic therapies can help control epilepsy, but any reduction in medication should be undertaken only under the guidance of a qualified health care professional.

Good to Know!
Warding Off a Seizure

If a seizure seems impending, there are a few things you can try to keep it from happening.

- Close your eyes, practice deep diaphragmatic breathing, and get into a relaxed state. You may want to visualize being in a beautiful tranquil state.
- If a particular smell seems to activate a seizure, try displacing that smell with another one. Some people have reported that the inhalation of essential oils such as lavender, clove, lemon, or orange can prevent a seizure.
- Change positions or move around. If there is another person around, have them grasp, shake, or tickle you to redirect the energy flowing through your neural pathways. (You might set up an agreement about this ahead of time with a family member so they know what to do.)
- Take two drops of Rescue Remedy under the tongue to calm yourself.

Nutritional Therapy

To minimize epileptic episodes, the diet should be high in fiber, with adequate protein. Eat lots of chlorophyll-rich foods, such as green leafy vegetables, as well as beans and whole grains. If you are taking Dilantin (phenytoin), which can cause a depletion of folic acid, increase your consumption of foods rich in folate (folic acid)—again, green leafy vegetables are a good option.

Eat small, frequent meals to help keep blood sugar levels stable. Abnormal blood sugar levels—whether too high or too low—can increase the likelihood of an epileptic seizure.

Skip This!

Avoid the following:

- Any foods you are sensitive to, as food allergies can be a causative factor in epileptic seizures.
- Sugar, refined carbohydrates, and alcohol, as these cause quick elevations in blood sugar, which then crash as the effects wear off.
- Aspartame, an artificial sweetener, which can increase seizures in people prone to them.
- Fried foods, which will only further obstruct the liver and heart.
- Mucus-forming foods, such fats, nuts and nut butters, hydrogenated oils, and concentrated sweets.
- Caffeine, which constricts blood vessels and can diminish blood supply to the brain.

Supplements for Well-Being

Vitamin B_6 is necessary for many factors essential to healthy brain function, such as the production of norepinephrine, as well as promoting calmness and energy. One rare form of epilepsy is due to a genetic requirement of large amounts of B_6 and so supplementing would be of extra importance. Be aware that B_6 can interfere with the absorption of the drug Dilantin.

Other supplements to consider include the following:

- **Calcium:** Needed for normal neurotransmission and relaxation.

- **Chromium (GTF):** Helps keep blood sugar levels and thus brain chemistry stable.

- **DMG (dimethylglycine):** Enhances oxygen utilization at a cellular level, so the brain gets the oxygen it needs.

◈ **GABA:** Anticonvulsant; can decrease excitatory messages to the brain.

◈ **Magnesium:** Naturally tranquilizing; can suppress electrical bursts in the brain.

◈ **Manganese:** Aids sugar metabolism, which is often deficient in those with epilepsy. Also normalizes neural activity.

◈ **Niacin:** Has a calming effect; when taken as a supplement for several months, it can decrease the need for anticonvulsant medicines.

◈ **Taurine:** Has a calming effect upon the nervous system. It helps stabilize nerve cell membranes and prevents neurons from producing excessive rapid impulses, which can lead to a seizure.

◈ **Vitamin E and selenium:** Should be taken after any traumatic head injury to help prevent brain damage from leading to epilepsy. Vitamin E may also help prevent seizures in children.

Healing Herbs

Throughout history, people have found various herbal remedies helpful in reducing seizures. Below are some to consider.

◈ **Bacopa:** In Ayurvedic medicine, bacopa is considered *medhya rasayan*, an herb that benefits the mind and spirit, and it has long been used to calm restlessness in children. It is a nourishing brain, nerve, and kidney tonic. It increases protein synthesis and brain-cell activity. It has also been found to help chelate heavy metals out of the body and heavy metal toxicity has sometimes been a factor in seizures.

◈ **Black cohosh:** For seizures associated with menses and after whooping cough. Relaxes chronic involuntary movements of the limbs and facial muscles and sedates the nerves, Antispasmodic, circulatory stimulant, nervine, sedative, and vasodilator.

- **Blue vervain:** For spastic nerve diseases; helps avert convulsions. Stimulates bile production, which moves liver stagnation. Antispasmodic, cholagogue, expectorant, nervine, and sedative.

- **Calamus:** Antispasmodic, cerebral stimulant, expectorant, nervine, sedative, and tonic.

- **Cannabis:** Contains cannabidiol (CBD), which can reduce seizures due to blocking excessive amplifying nerve signals.

- **Chickweed:** For inherited epilepsy and convulsions. Helps dissolve mucus. Rich in lecithin, which is nourishing to the brain. Nutritive.

- **Dandelion root:** Improves liver stagnation, clears heat and toxins from the blood, expectorant, and nutritive.

- **Gotu kola:** Antispasmodic, cerebral tonic, nervine, and peripheral vasodilator.

- **Lobelia:** Relaxes spasms by relaxing tissue, encourages deeper breathing, antispasmodic, nervine, and respiratory stimulant.

- **Mugwort:** Can be used in very small doses to gradually reduce the need for epilepsy medication (with guidance from a health care professional). Antispasmodic and nervine.

- **Oatstraw:** Nerve strengthening, relaxes spasms, nutritive for the brain and spinal cord, antispasmodic, cerebral tonic, nervine, and nutritive.

- **Passionflower:** Antispasmodic, nervine, and sedative. Enhances brain chemistry by calming the spirit, nourishing the central nervous system, and slowing down the breakdown of neurotransmitters. Used for hysteria and seizures (including grand mal).

- **Skullcap:** For twitches, convulsions, and grand mal seizures. Nourishes the brain and nerves, calms the heart, and quiets hysteria and excessive excitement. Antispasmodic, cerebral tonic, and nutritive.

- **Turmeric:** Moves liver stagnation and helps those who have been exposed to environmental pollutants.

- **Valerian:** For mild spasms, fainting spells, nervous anxiety, convulsions, trauma, and vertigo. Stimulates the release of GABA. Nervine, and sedative.

- **Wood betony:** For anxiety, catarrh, exhaustion, fear, hysteria, stress, and worry. Moves liver stagnation. Antispasmodic, cerebral tonic, liver tonic, nervine, and sedative.

Homeopathy

Homeopathic remedies that can be helpful for epilepsy include:

- **Argentum nitricum:** For nighttime seizures or those occurring with the menses or with emotional stress. For hand shaking and agitation after a seizure.

- **Cuprum metallicum:** For falling and foaming during seizure, with the thumbs flexing toward the palms.

- **Ferrum phosphoricum:** For seizures where blood rushes to the head.

- **Hydrocyanicum acidum:** For sudden violent convulsions, with cold extremities, rapid pulse, and weak heart.

- **Kali muriaticum:** A general remedy for epilepsy due to sluggish liver.

- **Kali phosphoricum:** For the person with epilepsy who feels cold after a seizure.

- **Natrum sulphuricum:** For epilepsy due to head injury.

🍃 **Nux vomica:** For hypersensitivity where the brain is overwhelmed by noise, light, and draft. For intense convulsions in which the spine and extremities bend forward.

🍃 **Silicea:** For nighttime seizures.

Mind-Body Therapies and Practices

It is essential to have your spine in alignment to minimize epileptic seizures. Consider craniosacral work, chiropractic adjustments, and osteopathic treatments.

Epilepsy can be a challenging condition to live with, and it can cause stress and even sometimes depression. Exercise can relax the body and help eliminate stress—good for the psyche and for the neuro-electrical system. Psychotherapy can help with any depression, as can any of the natural remedies discussed in chapter 5. Yoga is also helpful in these cases; postures that are especially beneficial for helping to prevent electrical short circuits in the brain include shoulder stands, backbends, and neck rolls. Deep slow breathing exercises (avoid rapid breathing exercises) and alternate nostril breathing can be very helpful in alleviating both stress and epilepsy. Avoid overly strenuous activity, and do your best to ward off fatigue and stress, which can worsen epilepsy.

On a daily basis, massage the feet, especially the big toe, which in reflexology corresponds to the head and brain. If you are comfortable with the idea, learn how to pull the big toe until it makes a gentle popping sound. Massage therapists or reflexologists can show you how to do this for yourself. Biofeedback, meditation, and behavioral conditioning can all be of help.

Hydrotherapy treatments are an ancient way to treat many conditions, including epilepsy, by using either hot or cold water to help direct blood toward or away from the various parts of the body. If an attack seems imminent, apply an ice pack to the head. Cold applications can also be given to the head after an attack. When showering direct a stream of cold water on the back of the neck at the end of the shower. The cold helps move stuck chi (including blood) away from the head region and helps resume circulation to the rest of the body.

Beneficial colors to use for epilepsy include indigo and violet to calm the motor nervous system and lemon yellow to support nerve transmission if poor brain circulation is a factor and one needs to invigorate.

As a general rule, epilepsy is best managed with regularity. Regularity of meals, exercise, and rest will all contribute to better brain stability.

10
Multiple
Sclerosis

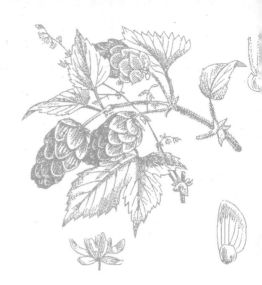

Multiple sclerosis (MS) is a neurodegenerative disease involving an autoimmune inflammatory reaction that can damage nerve fibers (axions) and break down the myelin sheath around nerves, leaving lesions.

In traditional Chinese medicine, MS is seen as a deficiency in the Liver or wood element, which governs the nerves, and cold and dampness in the kidneys and spleen, which depletes their vitality and leaves them deficient as well. It is considered a withering disease.

Natural remedies for MS are targeted toward protecting and rebuilding the myelin sheath, supporting the nervous system, normalizing immune function, reducing inflammation, improving circulation, and easing spasticity in muscles, as well as supporting the liver, kidneys, and spleen.

The earlier a patient begins a therapeutic program of nutritional and natural remedies in the treatment of MS, the more likely it is that they will experience benefits.

Nutritional Therapy

Foods to consider for MS are going to be anti-inflammatory, antioxidant, and energizing. It is also imperative to pay attention to the types of fats consumed. Brain tissue analysis of those with MS often shows higher-than-average levels of saturated fats, so avoid them. Be sure to avoid margarine, shortening, and other hydrogenated oils, as well as fried foods, potato chips, and the like. However, good-quality fats that are high in the anti-inflammatory compounds EPA and DHA are helpful for those with MS. Eat plenty of foods rich in omega-3 fatty acids, such as fatty fish—salmon, mackerel, sardines, herring—and flaxseed that help nerve cell function and myelin production and reduce nerve inflammation.

Other foods to eat more of include millet, nutritional yeast, and seaweeds. Vegetables to include are the nutritionally dense beets, cabbage, carrots, cauliflower, celery, and radishes. High-chlorophyll foods like green leafy vegetables, wheat grass, barley grass, kamut, chlorella, spirulina, and blue-green algae are energizing and helpful for balancing the immune system and delivering oxygen throughout the body. Include some fermented foods in the diet, like sauerkraut and kimchi to nourish the gut microbiome, where many brain chemicals originate. To aid digestion and improve circulation, include warming culinary herbs such as basil, black pepper, caraway, cinnamon, coriander, dill, fenugreek, ginger, mustard seed, rosemary, and sage.

Skip This!

As gluten can be inflammatory, a low-gluten diet has been found beneficial for MS; avoid wheat, rye, and barley. Do your best to stay off cow dairy products, which our systems are often intollerent to, and stimulants such as coffee. Be sure to avoid MSG (monosodium glutamate), aspartame, hydrolyzed vegetable protein, and similar additives, which are considered excitotoxins that overstimulate the nervous system.

Supplements for Well-Being

Beneficial supplements include the following.

- ● **Bromelain:** This enzyme derived from pineapple can reduce inflammation.

- ● **Enzymes:** Enzymes such as lipase and bile salts may help reduce circulating immune complexes that are damaging the myelin sheath.

- ● **Evening primrose, borage seed, and black currant seed oils:** These are good sources of omega-3 fatty acids, which can reduce nerve inflammation. They have been found to slow lymphocyte attacks upon the brain.

- ● **Lecithin:** Helps nourish the myelin nerve sheath.

- ● **Magnesium:** Can relax muscle spasms.

- ● **N-acetylcysteine (NAC) and liposomal glutathione:** Can help lower white blood cell levels, which can be elevated in people with MS.

- ● **Probiotics:** A probiotic supplement can improve digestion.

- ● **Vitamins B_2, niacin (B_3), and B_6:** All are needed for myelin formation.

- ● **Vitamin D:** Inhibits the production of interleukin-12, which is secreted by lymphocytes and involved in autoimmune disorders like MS. Vitamin D also stimulates the production of anti-inflammatory cytokines secreted by white blood cells.

- ● **Vitamin E and selenium:** Vitamin E helps reduce scarring—occurs when the myelin tissue is damaged—and selenium potentiates it.

Healing Herbs

Herbs can be used to improve circulation, provide the raw material to repair damage to the nervous system, and reduce inflammation.

🍃 **Arnica:** Moves congested blood. Used only externally and not on broken skin. Anti-inflammatory, immune stimulant, nerve stimulant, rubefacient, and vulnerary.

🍃 **Cannabis:** Cannabinoids have a neuroprotective effect, reducing inflammation and degeneration of the axions. Helps abate weakness, spasms, and depression associated with MS. Aids in balance and coordination, improves oxygen delivery to atrophied limbs, increases cerebral blood flow. Anticonvulsant, anti-inflammatory, and antispasmodic. A high-CBD strain will be most effective.

🍃 **Ginkgo:** Improves peripheral circulation, transmission of nerve signals, and brain function. For insufficient blood flow to legs, eye and ear problems, and dizziness. Antioxidant, cerebral tonic, circulatory stimulant, kidney tonic, and rejuvenative.

🍃 **Ginseng (Asian):** Nourishes the nervous system. Increases physical and mental alertness, helps the body adapt to stress, and relieves fatigue. Adaptogen, chi tonic, immune tonic, rejuvenative, restorative, and stimulant.

🍃 **Licorice root:** Improves energy and endurance. Chemically similar to though safer than cortisone. Adrenal tonic, anti-inflammatory, antispasmodic, chi tonic, demulcent, emollient, nutritive, and rejuvenative.

🍃 **Oatstraw:** Aids convalescence, convulsions, debility, fatigue, and stress. Antispasmodic, cerebral tonic, nerve tonic, nervine, nutritive, and rejuvenative.

🍃 **Saint John's wort:** Helps heal physically damaged nerves. Reduces pain by inhibiting serotonin breakdown. Alterative, anodyne, anti-inflammatory, antispasmodic, nervine, sedative, and vulnerary. Can be used internally and topically.

🍃 **Skullcap:** Nourishes brain and spinal cord and moves chi. Calms pain by reducing nerve excitability, improves motor coordination, relieves twitching and shaking, and is thought to help rebuild the myelin nerve sheath. Sometimes used to ease restlessness. Alterative, anodyne, antispasmodic, cerebral tonic, nervine, and sedative.

🍃 **Turmeric:** Reduces inflammation, including COX-2-related inflammation.

Chinese Patent Medicine

A Chinese patent formula to consider is Chen Pu Hu Chien Wan (Jian Bu Hu Qian Wan). It strengthens the kidneys, liver, and blood. It can help those with difficulty walking.

Homeopathy

A number of homeopathic remedies can help with MS.

🍃 **Arsenicum album:** For burning pain in the lower limbs, extreme thirst, and restlessness, when symptoms are worse from warmth and better after midnight and when cool.

🍃 **Causticum:** For when the right side of the body is more affected, and paralysis affects specific body parts, such as the face. For those who are thirsty and fear darkness and death.

🍃 **Conium maculatum:** For those whose legs are uncoordinated but pain-free; for paralysis; for those who are dizzy even when lying down and fear falling.

🍃 **Kali phosphoricum:** For weakness in the extremities, fatigue, pain, and prolapse of eye, with symptoms made worse by exertion.

🍃 **Lathyrus sativus:** For spastic paralysis, rigid legs, constant yawning, and fatigue.

🍃 **Magnesia phosphorica:** For painful spasms, twitching, eyes that are fatigued and hot. Vision may be blurred, and one may see colored objects before the eyes. Symptoms are made worse by warmth and pressure.

- **Nux vomica:** For when the left side of the body is more affected; the lower limbs, bladder, and anus may be affected, the face may be numb. The patient may experience twitching and irritabliity, may appear drunk, and may have difficulty swallowing.

- **Phosphorus:** For when paralysis ascends and the left side of the body is more affected. For weakness in the knees, bladder, and anus, a tendency to drop things, spaciness, and seeing spots and lights in front of the eyes.

- **Physostigma venenosum:** For those who walk as if drunk, with rigid muscles. Limbs may jerk when falling asleep.

- **Plumbum metallicum:** For painful paralysis and emaciation of the affected parts. The big toe may be painful. Symptoms are worse at night.

- **Strychninum phosphoricum:** For stiffness, twitching, weak spine, achiness, and burning sensations.

Flower Essences

Two flower essences show particular promise in the treatment of MS:

- **Gentian:** For those who are easily discouraged and pessimistic. For convalescence.

- **Gorse:** For feelings of hopelessness. For those who feel there is no reason to try but are being prodded on by friends and family. They won't be too excited about flower essences but may use them to please someone else. For depression brought on by chronic illness.

Mind-Body Therapies and Practices

Massage can be beneficial, especially when attention is paid to the back to increase circulation to the spinal cord. When getting massages, ask your therapist to massage you with olive oil; though it is stronger smelling than the lighter oils massage therapists usually use, it can be a good nourishing tonic. Adding some oil infused with St. John's wort would be excellent. A few drops of essential oil of lavender can be used to scent the oil and benefit the immune system. Foot reflexology can also be helpful, as can acupuncture.

Cool compresses can be applied to spastic muscles. This is best followed by exercise, optimally in the open air. Yoga, qigong, t'ai chi, and swimming (in unchlorinated water) are all excellent forms of exercise for someone with MS. The deep breathing and good posture they promote enable chi to flow more freely through the body.

Warm baths can also be helpful in relaxing muscles and nerves and stimulating circulation. Try infusing your bath with arnica flowers or thyme; tie up the herbs in a washcloth, place them in the tub with hot running water, and when the tub is filled to the desired level, turn off the water and let the bath cool as the flowers steep. When the temperature is appropriate, bathe, using the herb bundle to wash your body.

When showering, alternate the water temperature several times during its course, always starting warm and ending with cold, to encourage circulation and lymph flow. Practice dry brushing the skin for the same effect.

Colors to use in MS therapy include green for muscle strength, blue for its cooling qualities, scarlet for collagen production and tissue regeneration, and lemon yellow to decongest any blockage in and stimulate the motor nervous system. Crystals and sound therapy may also be helpful. Chanting can move energy blockages in the body and invigorate the brain and spinal column.

11
Parkinson's Disease

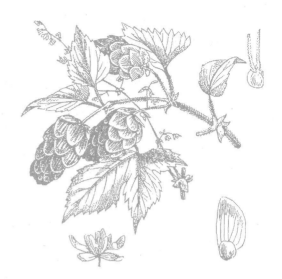

Parkinson's is a degenerative disease of the central nervous system. It manifests as uncontrollable movements, such as tremors, as well as stiffness and loss of balance, eventually leading to difficulty talking and walking.

In terms of natural remedies, helping the liver to better detoxify is imperative, as is reducing inflammation in the body.

Nutritional Therapy

A deficiency of dopamine is one causative factor for Parkinson's, and the disease is often treated with levodopa, a compound that is converted to dopamine in the brain. Fava beans also contain levodopa; add them to your diet to help your body produce dopamine. Mucuna beans are another option; they also contain levodopa.

Consume lots of raw green leafy vegetables and black seed *(Nigella sativa)* oil, and drink the fresh green leaves of cannabis as a juice to fortify the nervous system. (Note: cannabis is not psychoactive when raw, only when heated.)

Skip This!

It is important to decrease sugary foods and refined carbohydrates. Though this is important for everyone's health, when protecting brain health it becomes even more important so that you can fully optimize the nutrition you are taking in to nourish the healthy brain function. Toxins from environmental pollutants (especially heavy metals like mercury), food additives, and pharmaceuticals should all be considered as potential contributors to Parkinson's; do your best to avoid them.

Supplements for Well-Being

Supplements can reduce brain inflammation and help provide the raw material for proper neurotransmitter production and function.

- **Essential fatty acids:** Can inhibit prostaglandins that cause inflammation; try supplementing with sources such as evening primrose oil.

- **L-methionine:** Appears to be as effective as levodopa treatment and brings about further improvement in patients who have peaked in their recovery with allopathic medicine.

- **L-tyrosine:** Needed for the production of dopamine.

- **Niacin, folic acid, and vitamin B$_6$:** Can promote muscle coordination.

- **Phenylalanine:** Has been shown to improve the walking ability, muscle rigidity, speech impediments, and depression of patients with Parkinson's within a month.

- **Vitamins C and E:** Large doses of these vitamins have been shown to slow the progression of Parkinson's.

Healing Herbs

Herbs that can benefit people with Parkinson's disease include the following.

- **Ashwaghanda:** Helps with anxiety, fatigue, forgetfulness, memory loss, and tremors. Antispasmodic, nutritive, rejuvenative, and sedative.

- **Astragalus:** Contains some levodopa. Chi tonic.

- **Corydalis:** Reduces palsy and tremors. Antispasmodic and sedative.

- **Ginkgo:** Helps protect the brain from the damaging effects of Parkinson's disease.

- **Gotu kola:** Antispasmodic, cerebral tonic, nervine, rejuvenative, and vasodilator.

- **Oatstraw:** For anxiety, convulsions, and debility. Cerebral tonic, nerve tonic, nervine, nutritive, and rejuvenative.

- **Rhodiola:** Stimulates dopamine production in the brain. Improves brain cell activity and enables the brain to better utilize oxygen.

- **Rosemary:** For headache, stress, and vertigo. Antioxidant, antispasmodic, cholagogue, circulatory stimulant, nervine, rejuvenative, and tonic.

- **Saint John's wort:** Helps elevate dopamine levels. Antispasmodic, cholagogue, nervine, and sedative.

- **Skullcap:** Helps reduce tremors. Antispasmodic, cerebral tonic, nervine, and spinal tonic.

Mind-Body Therapies and Practices

Practice aerobic exercise to get more oxygen into the system and improve circulation. Qigong is another excellent practice as it promotes slow fluid movements that help a person with Parkinson's relax their body and move in a more flowing way. Regular massages are beneficial in tremor relief; use nervine essential oils, such as chamomile and rosemary, in the massage oil. Also consider acupuncture to lessen tremors, improve balance, and ease muscle rigidity.

12
Stroke and
Brain Injury

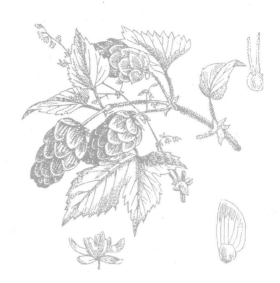

We hope that our mental faculties will always be functioning throughout our life, however stroke, medications, accidents, and traumas can all cause injury to our brain, causing our abilities to be impaired. Anything that inhibits the oxygen-rich blood from getting to the brain can cause impairment, whether a stroke or trauma to the head or body. Elevated levels of excess poor quality fats can contribute to blockages of oxygen delivering blood to the brain, so keeping cholesterol in check is a good preventive measure.

An ischemic stroke, which is the most common, occurs when a blood clot is the reason for blocking circulation to the brain. A hemorrhagic stroke results when an artery in the brain leaks or ruptures. Addressing high blood pressure early on is imperative to avoid this type of stroke. There is also a transient ischemic stroke, sometimes referred to as a mini-stroke, where blood flow to the brain is only blocked for less than five minutes.

It is important to recognize some of the symptoms of stroke as early action can reduce long term impairment:

- ▸ dizziness
- ▸ severe headache, especially in one who rarely gets headaches
- ▸ visual disturbances

- ▸ loss of balance and inability to walk or have coordination
- ▸ inability to comprehend
- ▸ facial numbness or weakness, especially on one side of the body

A head injury does not necessarily mean a brain injury. However, even though the skull protects the soft pliable mass of the brain, a sharp blow, shaking, rapid head or neck movements, or injury that causes bleeding and blood clots can cause pressure on the brain resulting in brain injury. After one has undergone proper medical screening and treatment, there are some things that can support one's recovery.

Nutritional Therapy

To facilitate recovery from a stroke or brain injury, begin with nourishing, easy-to-digest foods like soft cooked rice, oatmeal, baked winter squashes and sweet potatoes, unsweetened applesauce, yogurt, and miso soup, as a person's appetite is likely to be diminished. Miso soup and yogurt will additionally help replenish your system with friendly intestinal flora to strengthen your overall wellbeing on the road to recovery. Pureed vegetable and grain soups are a way of getting a variety of nutrients without having to serve lots of different dishes to a person who has a decreased appetite. Baked winter squashes and sweet potatoes are filling and nutrient rich.

If you are concerned about the possibility of blood clots, as you might be after a stroke, try eggplant; regular consumption of this vegetable has been shown to help dissolve blood clots.

Drink lemon in water and eat plenty of garlic to help prevent the blood from clumping together so nutrients can be delivered to the brain. Strengthen the blood vessels with flavonoids from plentiful fruits and vegetables, to help prevent rupturing of the arteries.

Eat some bioflavonoid rich foods such as blueberries and rose hip jam for their capillary strengthening abilities.

Supplements for Well-Being

When a brain injury has occurred, there are nutrients to support and speed recovery.

- **Acetyl-l-carnitine:** Research is showing that this can help prevent mental decline and improve learning ability.

- **Alpha-lipoic acid:** Can help protect the brain and nerve tissue and prevent free radical damage.

- **Bromelain:** An enzyme derived from pineapple that can aid in the reduction of traumatic swelling, inflammation, and pain.

- **Lecithin:** Lecithin helps lower serum cholesterol levels by breaking down fat and cholesterol. It is a naturally occuring component of the brain and a precursor of choline, which helps to form the neurotransmitter acetylcholne that supports healthy cognition, brain function, and structure.

- **Niacin (vitamin B$_3$):** Niacin increases cardiac output and dilates blood vessels, thus decreasing resistance in the circulatory system. Prolonged use of niacin lowers cholesterol. Note that niacin supplements can sometimes cause a hot, prickly sensation that lasts about ten minutes. Excessive use of niacin has the potential to irritate the liver. The timed-release versions of niacin are not effective and may be hepatotoxic.

- **Omega-3s:** The omega-3 fatty acids found in flaxseed oil, fish oil, evening primrose oil, and other sources (see page 306) can lower cholesterol, reduce blood pressure, and lower the risk of thrombosis (clot formation).

- **Vitamin A:** Works as an antioxidant, promotes the repair of epithelial tissue, and can help prevent infections from trauma or surgery as well as normalize white blood cell counts.

- **Vitamin C:** Vitamin C can help promote wound healing and prevent the buildup of deposits in the blood, relax blood vessel walls, and decrease the risk of blood clotting. It is a natural chelating agent and helps stimulate the production of lipoprotein lipase, an enzyme that dissolves fat on the arterial walls.

- **Vitamin E:** This vitamin improves HDL levels, reduces the "stickiness" of blood, and protects against the formation of blood clots. It also can help dissolve existing blood clots, reduce the risk of arteriosclerosis, prevent excessive scarring of the heart after a heart attack, and reduce angina. As a bonus, both internally and externally, it can help reduce any external scarring associated with the trauma or related injuries and can be used topically if any sutures were needed once they have been removed.

- **Zinc:** Promotes tissue repair and improved immune function for overall recovery after a traumatic brain injury or stroke.

Mother Nature's News

The amino acid methionine is a natural free radical scavenger and chelating agent that is being investigated for reducing stroke risk. Studies show that it can help lower homocysteine levels, which when levels are high can lead to stroke.

Healing Herbs

Herbs can provide concentrated nutrition, improve circulation, and promote regeneration of damaged tissues.

- **Cannabis:** Cannabidiol (CBD) constituents can help preserve and regenerate nerve cells and foster neuroplasticity.

- **Chaga mushroom:** A restorative that reduces neuroinflammation and facilitates cognition.

- **Ginger:** If nausea is a symptom either from injury or from anesthesia if surgeries are required, ginger can help allay this.

- **Ginkgo:** Improves neural transport.

- **Hawthorn:** Helps strengthen the cardiac force of the heart so that oxygen is delivered throughout the body, including the brain.

- **Lion's mane mushroom:** An adaptogen; promotes nerve regeneration by stimulating nerve growth factor (NGF), which can improve muscle-motor response pathways and support recovery from neurological trauma.

- **Red yeast rice (Monascus purpurens):** An ancient fermented fungal strain that grows from rice and helps decrease cholesterol, thus decreasing the risk of blood flow impairment to the brain.

- **Turmeric:** Helps reduce inflammation and reduce pain.

Chinese Patent Medicine

A Chinese patent formula that is used to improve blood flow, restore nerves, relieve pain, and improve range of motion is Xiao Yao Wan, which is targeted toward relieving liver stagnation. Another remedy to consider is Die Da Yao Jing, or Traumatic Injury Medicine Essence, which helps reduce pain and swelling.

Homeopathy

Natrum sulphuricum is helpful in activating healing of head injuries where mental capabilities have been impaired. Homeopathic arnica can be taken after a brain trauma or related surgery to aid in reducing swelling and pain.

Flower Essences

Rescue Remedy can be an excellent ally after a traumatic brain injury or stroke. Emotions that are unexpected and sometimes irrational are likely to occur and can be part of the healing process, Rescue Remedy can help sooth these.

Aromatherapy

Both calamus essential oil and rosemary essential oil help support restoration of memory function after trauma. The lavender essential oil is both uplifting and antiseptic, which can be useful if recovering in a hospital room or rehab facility. They can be diffused in a room.

Mind-Body Therapies and Practices

Chiropractic work, craniosacral work, physical therapy, occupational therapy, and speech therapy can help improve blood flow, reduce pain, and help patients regain range of motion and other general functions.

Exercise of any form will help your brain reconnect with your body, so during recovery, do some form of exercise every day, even if it is simply stretching your toes and fingers. A physical therapist can help you select the exercises that are specific for your condition or, when you can, stretching, swimming, and yoga can all be helpful, as can massage. But if that's too much for you, use Chinese hand balls, squeezy hand toys, and handheld gyroscopes.

Try the exercise of tightening your toes, then totally relaxing, then the feet, relax, then ankles, and you gradually move up the body. If you can't move your body as you wish, visualize yourself making those movements. Visualize sending healing energy, healing light, and healing colors into the parts of your body that need it. Give thanks for the things that are right in your life.

Write It Down (or Speak It Out)
Write, type, or record with your voice the story of your life or your accident. Just the act of putting it down on paper can be cathartic and healing and may even help you reveal new learning or a silver lining. Write

the story of how you want your future to look like—visualize your healing and put it down on paper/record it in your own words. How might you use this time of healing so that you emerge with new strength and vitality? In what ways do you want to regenerate and renew? And what might you need or want to start fresh?

Practical Tips for Recovery from Brain Injury,
Stroke, and Related Surgeries

Release. Screaming into a pillow for no more than ten minutes can be releasing and therapeutic if you feel a need for it during the recovery process.

Use music. Music during recovery and any subsequent operations can reduce anxiety and blot out noise pollution that could be detrimental. Assure that you hear what you need and want to hear.

Brighten your space. Whether you are at home or in a hospital or rehab facility, see if you can have your own colorful sheets or comfortable clothes or run an aromatherapy diffuser with a comforting scent to brighten your spirits. As noted, lavender essential oil can be uplifting and antiseptic. Displaying a piece of beautiful inspirational art in your line of site if you are mostly static will help your psyche feel inspired and comforted.

When it is time to get back on your feet, do it gradually, with care and moderation. Try to savor the taking of time for your own healing process!

13
ADHD

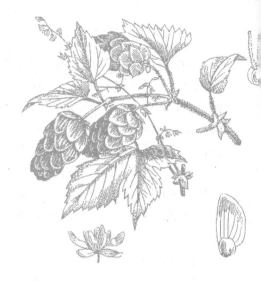

Attention deficit hyperactivity disorder (ADHD) and similar diagnoses are coming to be understood as neurodivergencies rather than disorders. ADHD manifests across a range of cognitive differences and defies the kind of specific categorization and labeling our culture tends to crave.

According to the U.S. Centers for Disease Control, over the years 9.8 percent of children in the United States have been diagnosed with attention deficit hyperactivity disorder (ADHD). There are many complementary and alternative remedies to address the more challenging aspects of ADHD.

Natural remedies can help ease some of the challenges of ADHD by enhancing focus and memory and calming the nerves.

Nutritional Therapy

One of the most common exacerbating factors in ADHD and the easiest to change is diet. Any foods that are stimulating or inflammatory can contribute to issues with attention and hyperactivity. For this reason, you may wish to avoid sugar, hydrogenated oils, artificial colorings and flavorings, nitrates, caffeine and other stimulants, and any foods that are highly processed and can contribute to inflammation, including of the brain. As a general rule, avoid any foods that contribute to a blood sugar rush, such as sodas and even fruit juices, which can put one on a roller coaster ride of mood changes. You may also wish to check for food allergies or sensitivities, as digestive issues and allergic reactions will cause irritation and inflammation in the body. Wheat, dairy, eggs, tomatoes, corn, soy, peanuts, shellfish, citrus, and yeast are common allergens; practice a food elimination diet and keep a food journal to determine what the culprit may be.

Traditional Chinese medicine often considers ADHD as an overly heated condition, and cooling foods, such as green leafy vegetables, celery, and cucumbers, can be helpful. Blue and purple fruits and vegetables are a good source of anthocyanins, which support microcirculation in the brain so the brain is able to receive all of the nutrients and oxygen it requires and promote alertness.

Omega-3 essential fatty acids help overall brain development and function. Wild salmon and sardines are well known for their omega-3 content. Raw tahini, walnuts, seaweeds, and chia, hemp, and flaxseeds are good vegan sources.

Enzymes in fresh raw food can help reduce brain inflammation (as well as any other inflammation in the body), so uncooked fruits and vegetables can be helpful. If using soy, choose fermented soy such as miso, tempeh, and tamari instead of tofu and soy milk, as they are less inflammatory, as anything one is sensitive to can cause inflammation in the sinuses, skin, and joints, but also the brain. Brain inflammation can be a contributing factor in many cases of ADHD.

Since avoiding irritants is one of the goals of ADHD therapy, eat organic as much as possible to minimize the amount of chemicals you are exposed to. Drink plenty of pure water to help the body eliminate toxins.

Supplements for Well-Being

A range of supplements can benefit those with ADHD, including the following.

- **Calcium and magnesium:** Have muscle-relaxing properties and aid sleep. Magnesium also calms overexcitability.

- **B-complex vitamins:** Can have a calming effect. They also improve neurotransmission and improve appetite.

- **GTF chromium:** Helps keep blood sugar levels stable and decreases sugar cravings.

- **Digestive enzymes:** These enzymes, such as bromelain, papain, and pancreatin, can help reduce inflammation and calm moods.

- **GABA:** Helps protect the brain from bombardments of excitatory, anxiety-related messages. It has a very tranquilizing effect, calming anxiety without causing sedation.

- **Omega-3:** As noted, omega-3s provide food for overall brain health.

Make sure any supplements you take are free of artificial colorings and flavorings as they can exacerbate the symptoms.

Healing Herbs

Herbs that can help people with ADHD include the following:

- **Bacopa:** Increases attention span, memory, learning capacity, and motor coordination. It enhances the ability to learn new tasks and aids in the retention of newly learned material. Bacopa raised IQ scores in a twelve-week study of hyperactive children.

- **Catnip:** Relaxes the nerves and calms anxiety, hysteria, insomnia, and restlessness.

- **Chamomile:** A gentle relaxant that tones the nervous system, which can be helpful for those prone to temper tantrums. It helps restore an exhausted nervous system and relaxes muscles.

- **Ginkgo:** Enhances cerebral blood flow, calms anxiety, and reduces memory loss. It increases the uptake of glucose and improves nerve signal transmission and neurotransmitter function.

- **Guarana:** Helps build focus and attention and can help calm excessive motor activity, much the same way as Ritalin (which is a stimulant for adults, but sedative for children). Since it contains caffeine, use it only in small amounts.

- **Kava kava:** Relaxes the muscles without numbing one's mental focus.

- **Lemon balm:** Protects the cerebrum from excessive stimuli. It calms anxiety and relieves depression, hysteria, insomnia, nervousness, restlessness, and nightmares.

- **Oatstraw and milky oats:** Calm and nourish the nervous system.

- **Passionflower:** Quiets the central nervous system and slows the breakdown of neurotransmitters. It is an herb of choice to relieve anger, anxiety, hyperactivity, hysteria, irritability, insomnia, muscle spasms, restlessness, rapid speech, and stress.

- **Valerian:** A strong central nervous system relaxant. It can help improve concentration for those under stress. It calms aggressive behavior, anxiety, delirium, hyperactivity, hysteria, insomnia, nervous breakdown, nervousness, restlessness, and stress and can help counteract the effects of shock and trauma.

Calming herbal baths can provide centering and relaxation. A few of the above herbs can be tied into a "lost sock" and steeped in a hot bath as a way of taking in the herb's properties. Consider for this catnip, oats, or lemon balm.

Flower Essences

Flower essences to consider using include:

- **Chestnut Bud:** For those who make the same mistakes repeatedly.

- **Clematis:** For those who daydream excessively.

- **Gentian:** For those who give up easily.

- **Larch:** For those who lack confidence.

- **White Chestnut:** To dispel persistent unwanted thoughts.

- **Wild Rose:** For those who lack motivation.

Aromatherapy

Those with ADHD can benefit from aromatherapy through the opening of neural pathways and its immediate ability to affect consciousness in a gentle and pleasant way. Include lavender, orange, peppermint, and rosemary, which can aid concentration. Diffuse them in a room. Add five drops to a warm bath. Or take five deep inhalations from the bottle with each nostril.

Mind-Body Therapies and Practices

People with ADHD tend to do best in an environment that is calm and clear. Noise, clutter, visual distractions, and disruptions can lead to overstimulation and difficulty with attention and retention, with the potential for irritability, impulsivity, hyperactivity, and even hostility. Make your home a mellow, calm environment. Strive for a schedule of regularity—regular meals, regular activity, and regular sleep schedule. Clear clutter from your home; strive for organization and good feng shui. Provide soft natural lighting. Keep your bedroom free of electromagnetic pollution. Minimize time with TV, video games, and other electronics. Clean the house of environmental toxins such as smoke, molds, and chemical fumes.

Exercise is helpful for releasing energy and calming the nervous system, not to mention supporting overall health. Spending time out in nature has a similar effect, so get outside—gardening, hiking, biking, and swimming are excellent activities. A martial arts practice can help develop focus and provide an outlet for energy.

Practical Tips for ADHD

Engage physically. Physical contact such as hugging and massage can stimulate calming endorphin production.

Try craniosacral work. It can help relieve energy to flow unrestricted to the brain by improving energetic and physical alignment.

Try neurofeedback or biofeedback. It can help train the brain's ability to function optimally and help the body and brain process stressful situations.

Try a craft. An easy portable craft can help engage the brain when one must sit still.

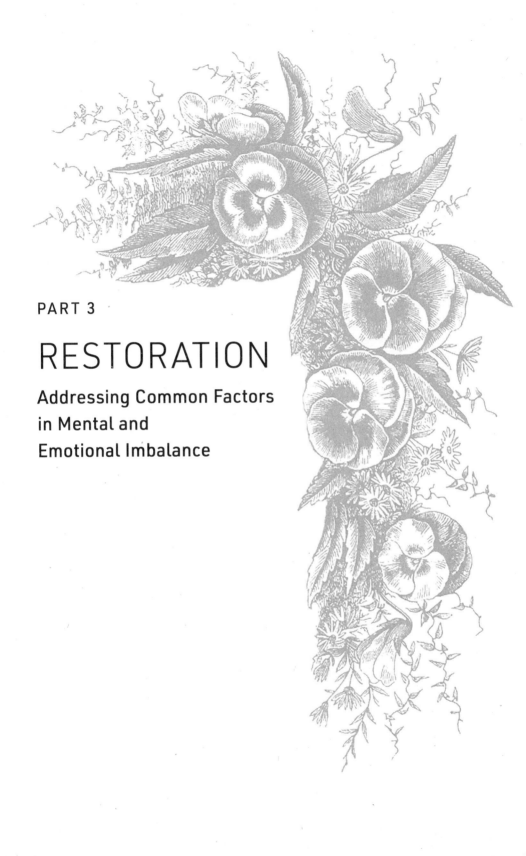

PART 3

RESTORATION

Addressing Common Factors
in Mental and
Emotional Imbalance

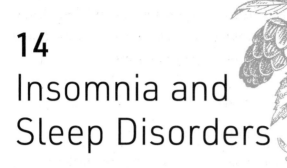

14
Insomnia and Sleep Disorders

Blissful sleep is that recharging, rejuvenating repose in which we spend about one-third of our lives. When we rest, our bone marrow and lymph nodes produce substances that aid the immune system, and much of the body's repair work is done. Yet for many, sleep can be elusive, leaving them exhausted and lacking mental clarity the next day.

Lack of quality sleep lessens our emotional resiliency, making us feel less than able to meet each day's challenges and more likely to experience upset over minor and major events. When we sleep well, we are able to meet the day. The best way to improve sleep is to address the cause.

Reasons Why You Can't Sleep

What you do, think, eat, and drink can determine whether or not you get the sleep you need. Caffeinated foods and beverages such as coffee, black tea, chocolate, and cola drinks, even when consumed early in the day, can affect normal night sleep patterns. Alcohol consumption interferes with deep REM (rapid eye movement) sleep. Nicotine is a stimulant, and smokers can take longer to fall asleep than nonsmokers.

Many prescription medications contribute to insomnia, including antibiotics, cold remedies, decongestants, steroids, appetite suppressants, contraceptives, and thyroid pills. Allergies, pain, anxiety, and depression can all interfere with sleep. But sleeping pills can inhibit calcium absorption, are often habit forming, and can prevent dreaming, and thus should not be a first resort for sleeping problems.

Good to Know!

If needing to use the bathroom awakens you, try elevating your feet and practicing toe and heel lifts during the day to help the body absorb fluids that would otherwise go through the kidneys at night.

Nutritional Therapy

Turkey, tuna, whole-grain crackers and bread, nut butters, bananas, grapefruits, avocados, dates, and figs all contain tryptophan, an amino acid that promotes the production of serotonin, a chemical in the brain that induces sleep. Try eating a tryptophan-rich snack an hour before bedtime.

Skip This!

Some foods can actually disrupt sleep because they contain the amino acid tyramine, which discourages the production of serotonin; these include cheese, spinach, sauerkraut, ham, sausage, bacon, and dark chocolate (which also contains caffeine). Many members of the nightshade family, such as tomatoes, potatoes, eggplant, and bell peppers, also interfere with sleep because their alkaloid solanine can disrupt calcium assimilation, and when calcium levels are low, that can contribute to insomnia.

In women, insomnia can be caused by hormonal influences, such as when you have bloating from premenstrual syndrome (PMS). For women experiencing PMS it can be important to avoid extra salt to prevent fluid retention, to skip caffeine to prevent mineral depletion, and to take extra calcium and magnesium to relax the muscles and promote a state of calm. For a bedtime snack, try a soy smoothie. Soy is a plant estrogen source, and milk contains sleep-inducing tryptophan, so it's a good combo.

Supplements for Well-Being

A calcium and magnesium supplement can be helpful when taken before bed, as it has a muscle-relaxing, calming effect. The body also best absorbs calcium when at rest.

B vitamins such as B_3 (niacin) and B_6 (pyridoxine) help produce the body's natural sleep chemicals—tryptophan and serotonin. Take them forty-five minutes before you go to bed; otherwise, they can overstimulate the body's deep sleep (REM) cycle and actually disrupt sleep.

Theanine promotes sleep and improves immune function. 5-HTP helps the body make calming serotonin. Theanine, 5-HTP, and inositol are particularly helpful for those who have trouble staying asleep.

Healing Herbs

Unlike potent pharmaceutical sleep aids, the herbs that promote good sleep are usually not habit forming and don't leave you feeling groggy. Here are the ones to try.

- **Chamomile:** Its antispasmodic properties help you unwind from tension.

- **Hops:** Contain lupulin, a strong yet safe, reliable sedative. Even the aroma of hops can help lull you to sleep. In fact, hops can be made into a sleep sachet (a five-by-five-inch) pouch stuffed with dried hops, stitched up, and placed in your pillowcase). Both King George II and Abraham Lincoln are said to have slept with hops pillows. Make a new sachet twice a year.

- **Passionflower:** Slows the breakdown of serotonin and norepinephrine, helping you to move into a more peaceful state of consciousness and calming anxiety.

- **Skullcap:** Contains scutellarin, which transforms into scutellarein in the body and stimulates the brain to produce calming endorphins.

- **Valerian:** Calms sleep disorders that result from anxiety.

- **Wild lettuce:** A powerful sleep aid.

All of the above herbs can be taken by themselves or in combination, before you go to bed or during the night, whether as teas, tinctures, or capsules.

If you tend to wake up during the night, place a glass with just a bit of water by your bed so that you can squeeze a dropperful of herbal tincture into it and drink it. This is the easiest way to use herbs to help you get back to sleep, and the least likely to cause you to be awakened later by the urge to urinate.

Aromatherapy

Adding essential oils to a warm bath before bed can be a wonderfully relaxing sleeping aid. After the tub has filled, add seven drops of calming essential oil of chamomile or lavender for their relaxing effects. Another technique is to put two or three drops of chamomile or lavender oil on the pillowcase, so you inhale their calming scent when you need to sleep. You can also try lemon balm, marjoram, neroli, nutmeg, rose, sandalwood, and ylang-ylang.

Mind-Body Therapies and Practices

We all know that some things in life are outside of our control. But there are many things we can do for our bodies as well as in our environments to set ourselves up for a good night's rest.

Good to Know!

Research shows that inadequate vasodilation, the opening of blood vessels to increase blood flow, may cause sleep problems. That's because when we lie down, the body lowers its core temperature and redistributes heat to the periphery. To remedy this problem, just tuck a hot water bottle near your feet or slip on a pair of cozy socks to help regulate the body's core temperature, relaxing and widening blood vessels that constrict when it's cold, which can keep you awake.

Get Enough Sun

Sunlight is the most powerful regulator of our biological clock, influencing when we feel sleepy and when we feel alert. So a lack of light exposure can result in difficulty sleeping. If you have trouble falling asleep, spend some time outside in the early morning sunlight, even on cloudy days. Try taking a walk outside for forty-five minutes. Or just sit outside for forty-five minutes; all you really need is for your eyes to bathe in natural light. If sunlight isn't available, consider a light box or light visor.

Exercise for Better Sleep

Exercise can have a huge impact on the quality of your sleep. In a study reported in the *Journal of the American Medical Association* in 1997, Stanford researchers placed a group of sedentary people with sleep problems on a program of moderate exercise. After sixteen weeks, the exercisers were getting to sleep twice as fast and were sleeping more than forty minutes longer each night.

Although exercise can aid sleep, some studies suggest that exercising too close to bedtime does just the opposite. This is because exercise causes your body to feel awake, alert, and energized, and it raises body temperature. But if you exercise five or six hours before you go to bed, and your temperature has had time to drop, you'll find you sleep easier.

Establish a Sleep Routine

You'll sleep better if you set regular bed and awakening times and do your best to stick with them. Make the hour to two hours before you go to bed a wind-down period from the day's activities and stresses. Read or watch television in a room other than your bedroom so the body knows the bedroom is reserved for sleep. Avoid excessive mental stimulation right before bed, such as action-packed TV or page-turning novels. Try holistic practices such as taking a hot bath or doing some self-massage (or, even better, getting a massage) before going to sleep. Sex, too, can be a pleasurable prelude to sleep.

Make Your Bedroom a Peaceful Sanctuary

Keep your bedroom space serene and avoid using it as a place to do homework, pay bills, conduct business, or carry out arguments. Keep your sleeping environment quiet, dark, cool, and safe. The bedroom should ideally be a calm color, such as blue. Keep the bedroom between 60°F and 66°F. Allow a bit of fresh air into the bedroom at night (unless you are using an air purifier), though not directly by the head. Put your bed in the quietest, darkest corner of the room. Make your bed as comfy as possible. If you can, use natural bedding, such as organic sheets and blankets, to allow your skin to breathe. Set the alarm clock and hide it where you can't see it to prevent the anxiety that can result when you can't sleep and keep looking at the clock.

Avoid Environmental Allergens

Environmental allergies can interfere with sleep and contribute to stuffy noses and headaches in the morning. To minimize allergens in your bedroom, wash bedding in hot water (130°F) every week to kill dust mites, the microscopic organisms that feed off flakes of dead skin. A dehumidifier, a high-efficiency particulate air filter, and zippered, allergen-proof covers on your bedding and blankets can all help you sleep easier.

Good to Know!

Electromagnetic pollution too close to the body can stimulate the nervous system and weaken the immune system. So avoid having clocks, stereos, and electric blankets as your nighttime companions within 6 feet of your bed.

Dim the Lights

Remember that light is a stimulant. If streetlights shine brightly through your windows at night, consider getting heavier curtains. If you awake during the night and need to go to the bathroom, avoid turning on bright lights, as this will make you even more awake and inhibits the melatonin production needed for sleep. Instead, use a small red nightlight to guide your way. Avoid checking your phone in the night; the blue light it emits will only aggravate any sleep issues. If needed, use earplugs or eye masks to help shut out the world out for a while. Eye masks are a must for Brigitte (especially after teaching in Iceland during bright summer nights)!

Quiet Your Mind

If you have too much on your mind, like plans for the days ahead, things to do, and people to call, write it all down and then let it all go. This makes it easier to relax, rather than needing to lie awake and review your to-do list. If you are troubled about something, try to talk about your feelings with someone you trust.

Focus on Your Breath

When you are ready to go to bed, try focusing on the in and out of your breath to soothe yourself to sleep. Couple breathing with some sort of visualization. For example, with one breath relax your toes, with the next breath your feet, then your ankles; moving slowly up your body should help you slumber. By the time you reach your waist you might very well be asleep! Or try counting backward from a high number, slowly, one number for each breath.

Visualize Your Calm, Safe Place

Visualization can also help you to relax and ease you off to sleep. Try closing your eyes and using all of your senses; see yourself in a safe, calm place like the beach, a lake, or the woods. Or try listening to sleep visualization, meditation, or yoga nidra recordings to help you relax and drift off to sleep.

Write It Down

Keeping a sleep journal to track how each night's sleep went as well as your intake of caffeine, what you ate that day, and possible stressors can help you to locate the cause of your sleeplessness.

If You Just Can't Sleep

If you can't sleep for more than half an hour, don't fight it. Instead, get up and practice a quiet activity in a dimly lit room that won't rev you up, like reading (no thrillers!), knitting, or listening to calming music until you feel sleepy, and then return to bed.

If you have trouble sleeping, try not to focus on this fact during the day. Just get up in the morning, go through your day, and get into bed at your regular time. Try the strategies you've found here and you will sleep more easily!

Natural Secrets for Sweet Dreams

Dreams are a way of clearing the subconscious and may give us insight about what lies deep in our psyche. They usually last anywhere from a few moments to more than forty minutes. It is amazing how in just a few seconds we can traverse years of experience in these "fantasies of the night." At the very least, dreams can be an opportunity for adventure and entertainment.

Tricks and Tips for Sweet Dreams

A dream pillow is a sachet filled with herbs whose scent can help us access the deep parts of the mind and make dreams more vivid. Make a five-by-five-inch sachet filled with dried lavender, lemon balm, and rosemary. Place the sachet in your pillowcase when you go to bed. Make a new pillow or refill the original every six months.

Kava kava is another option; it is said to induce epic-length dreams worth remembering. Damiana can be smoked or taken as a bedtime tea for vivid dreams. Since damiana is also an aphrodisiac, dreams may be of an erotic nature. Saint John's wort is recommended in Europe to promote lucid dreams and help dispel nightmares. Burning jasmine incense before bed may help transport you to the Land of Dreams.

The amethyst is regarded as the stone for dreaming. Place some amethysts around the head of your bed to foster dreams.

Taking vitamin B_6 and zinc before you go to sleep can enhance your ability to recall your dreams.

Set Your Intention before You Go to Sleep

Before you go to sleep, remind yourself that you wish to remember your dreams. You can also set an intention ("my dreams will reveal wisdom") or ask for guidance on a particular issue. Keep asking. Your final thoughts of the day will often have an influence upon your life. It may be helpful to read something spiritually uplifting before bed to put you into a state of exploring consciousness.

Natural Practices for Remembering Sweet Dreams

The best time to try to recall your dreams is when you first wake up, but if you begin the day with an adrenaline rush produced by a shrill alarm clock, you'll have little chance of remembering them. Instead, try slowly waking up to a clock that plays soft music or Tibetan bells or a sunrise clock so that you have time for reflection. It is also possible to mentally program yourself to wake up a few minutes before the alarm ever goes off.

Once you are awake, try lying still with your eyes still closed. Let the images of your dreams drift into your consciousness.

Keep writing implements by the bed to record those flashes of recall. Every morning, write down something about your dreams. If you lack any recall, write, "Nothing remembered." The important factor is to get in the habit of writing something daily. (Alternatively, you could record yourself speaking about them.) If you can remember a feeling, but not the actual dream, try to think of what situation could bring up that feeling. It may facilitate remembering. Telling your dream to a friend may give you a bit more insight into its details and meaning.

A folk remedy to aid dream recall is to place a glass of water by the bed. Drink half the glass before going to sleep and the other half when you awaken.

Look up some of the symbols you dream about, even if it is just a brief remembrance of a color, person, mood, or image. You can find plenty of dream interpretation information online and in books. Enjoy the journey!

Dealing with Nightmares

According to traditional Chinese medicine, nightmares can correlate to organ deficiencies. Nightmares can be disturbing, but they get your attention, and you may want to explore what their significance is. For example:

- ► Dreaming of drowning or suffocating may indicate the lungs are overactive and need to be calmed.
- ► Dreams of crying can indicate lung deficiency.

- ▸ Dreams of failure, such as being unable to complete a task, may mean excess spleen/pancreas energy.
- ▸ Dreams of being rejected by loved ones may indicate a spleen/pancreas deficiency.

If the cardiovascular system is stressed and overworking, dreams of fire, explosives, and heat may occur. A person with a deficient heart may have dreams where they are unable to talk or scream.

Kidney excess may manifest as dreams of water and snakes. If the kidneys are depleted, the dreams are more fearful, such as being pursued by snakes or swept away by water. Liver excess can result in dreams of impatience, anger, and danger. Liver deficiency may bring dreams of indecision, doom, gloom, and even death.

Natural Remedies for Bad Dreams

Banish nightmares with calming basil, chamomile, dill seed, rosemary, and wood betony as these herbs promote deep rest and have long been used for calming the nerves. These herbs can be prepared as teas, wrapped up in sachets to tuck in your pillow, or hung as sprigs over the bed. Some find cannabis to be helpful, and for some people cannabis may decrease dreams in general.

Skip This

Rich, spicy, or oily foods as well as foods you are allergic to can provoke nightmares.

The flower essences Aspen, Rock Rose, and Rescue Remedy all help calm panic and prevent nightmares. Using the color violet in color therapy helps calm the spirit.

May all your best dreams come true!

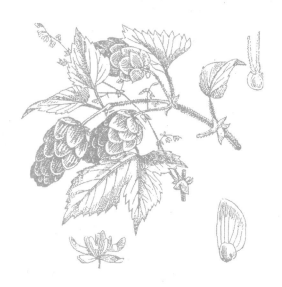

15
Fatigue

Are you tired of being tired? When you make your bed in the morning, do you feel like getting back into it? When you don't have enough energy, daily life becomes more difficult and can leave you feeling cranky and overwhelmed.

Before you try natural remedies, it's important to rule out any medical reasons for fatigue. Feeling tired can be a sign that you have a condition like hypothyroidism, chronic Lyme disease, hypoglycemia, anemia, a nutritional deficiency, or allergies. Talk to your health care practitioner about what tests you might need to determine the cause of your fatigue and how to treat it.

Once you've eliminated medical reasons for fatigue, it's time to explore natural remedies. When you need power in your house, for a lamp, TV, or computer, you plug a socket into an outlet. It's the same with the natural practices outlined here to relieve fatigue: We can plug into them to boost our energy. The first step is deciding which habits you want to adopt, whether it's using herbs, supplements, aromatherapy, exercise, or yoga. The next step is to practice them daily so energy is there when you need it.

Nutritional Therapy

To begin, check in with your nutrition to make sure you are getting adequate calories and good-quality proteins, carbohydrates, and fats, as well as sufficient vitamins and minerals. Try to make lunch the main meal of the day, as more energy is required midday than in the evening. Foods for sustained energy include seeds (pumpkin, sesame, sunflower, all soaked), nuts that are high in potassium (especially almonds), beans (a rich source of glucose, the body's preferred food), and fresh raw vegetables and fruit. Chia seeds provide stamina too, and they make an energizing breakfast. Avoid overeating as it just makes your body work harder. Both being undernourished and carrying around extra pounds can cause fatigue so food is an important ingredient to energy wellness!

Skip This!

Eating something you are sensitive or allergic to can make you feel foggy and groggy. Keeping a food journal can help you pinpoint which foods you're allergic to or even just which ones make you feel tired. Dairy products, wheat, gluten, yeast, citrus, and corn are common culprits. You'll be amazed by how much better you feel after eliminating any offending foods.

Additionally, if you can, avoid consuming microwaved food. It's not conducive to building the life energy and vitality you need.

Also avoid sugar and caffeine. While they may give you a quick high, you'll soon crash. That's because when insulin is produced to handle the sugar infusion, your blood sugar drops, leaving you feeling jittery and even more tired. Sugar and caffeine also deplete the body of needed nutrients for energy, such as vitamin B_{12} and calcium.

Go Green!

Green foods such as collards, dandelion greens, kale, spinach, violets, and supergreens like blue-green algae, spirulina, chlorella, barley grass, and wheatgrass are loaded with nutrients such as beta-carotene, iron, protein, and chlorophyll, the wonderful, oxygen-transporting lifeblood of plants. Mineral-rich sea vegetables such as dulse, kelp, and wakame are excellent foods for those whose fatigue is caused by or made worse by low thyroid function.

The Buzz on Bee Pollen

Bee pollen can be added to smoothies as an energy booster. If you have pollen allergies, however, start with tiny amounts (one-grain-a-day increments) and increase over a long period of time to 1 teaspoon daily, unless you find that bee pollen is not your ally.

Dark Chocolate

If you want a treat, eat dark chocolate. The theobromine in chocolate is a mild stimulant. Chocolate also contains phenylethylamine (PEA), which is a feel-good mood elevator. Choose high-quality, imported dark chocolate with 70 percent or more cacao content. It has less sugar, and its rich flavor will satisfy you with less. Aim for 1 ounce of dark chocolate a few times a week.

Energizing Drinks

Sipping small amounts of chilled water every thirty minutes sends a signal to your brain to increase alertness and energy. That's because drinking cold water stimulates an adrenaline release by activating the sympathetic nervous system, the same system that activates the fight-or-flight reaction.

If you've been sitting for too long, your body switches to the parasympathetic nervous system mode, which makes you calm but also can make you feel tired. Cold water will switch you back into the sympathetic side of the nervous system and wake you up.

Rehydration will increase your energy quotient too. If you don't have access to cold water in your workplace, keep cold water in the fridge at home and bring it to work in an insulated cup so you can "chill" all day long! Splashing your face with cold water will also increase energy because it, too, stimulates the release of adrenaline.

In addition to water, add green tea to your routine. It does contain some caffeine, but more importantly, it contains L-theanine, an amino acid that has a stress-reducing effect on your brain. It helps calm you down while leaving your mind clear, sharp, and alert.

Supplements for Well-Being

A vitamin B-complex supplement impacts brain function and energy levels and can help cover all the bases to ensure that no deficiencies are contributing to low energy.

Healing Herbs

The following herbs have traditionally been used to increase stamina. See if they work for you!

- ◢ **Ashwagandha:** Relieves lethargy and fatigue.

- ◢ **Dandelion root:** Increases vitality.

- ◢ **Ginkgo:** Helps the brain better utilize oxygen, improves mental alertness, and improves peripheral circulation.

- ◢ **Ginseng:** Relieves exhaustion, helps the body deal with stress, nourishes the adrenal glands, and reduces fatigue.

- ◢ **Licorice root:** Is naturally sweet, helps normalize blood sugar levels, and nourishes exhausted adrenal glands.

- ◢ **Schisandra berry:** Helps with endurance, fatigue, and insomnia.

- ◢ **Yerba maté:** Rich in minerals, as well as some caffeine. (This one has helped Brigitte write so many books!)

Flower Essences

Flower essences are a gentle way to put more sparkle in your step.

- ◢ **Hornbeam:** For those who feel overwhelmed by life.

⚕ **Olive:** Helps combat fatigue when you feel you have reached the end of your rope, daily activities seem difficult, and you wish only to sleep.

Aromatherapy

Certain essential oils can work to improve both physical and psychological energy levels. They include basil, clary sage, geranium, lavender, lemon, orange, and rosemary.

Peppermint can help wake you up, too. According to a study in the *North American Journal of Psychology*, drivers who were exposed to the scent of peppermint were more alert and had more energy. Consider chewing strong peppermint gum or enjoying peppermint mints during the day to decrease fatigue and increase alertness. Eucalyptus and spearmint have similar qualities to peppermint.

For the other essential oils, place a few drops on a tissue and inhale deeply, or simply take ten deep inhalations from the bottle. Washing your face with cold water and a drop of Dr. Bronner's peppermint soap can be very vivifying.

Mind-Body Therapies and Practices

From quick fixes to long-term and daily strategies here are ways to enhance energy and combat fatigue in your body and mind.

Acupressure
A good do-it-yourself practice to boost energy is acupressure on your outer ear. When you apply pressure to acupressure points all along the outer ear, it helps clear your head, gets rid of dull pain above the neck, and charges up your entire energy system. Just use your thumb and first finger to squeeze up and down the entire outer ear two or three times, giving it a good, brisk rubbing. This simple acupressure technique stimulates the energy in your whole body and gets it moving.

Deep Breathing

If your breathing is shallow, your brain may miss out on the recharging properties of oxygen—one of life's free remedies! Oxygen nourishes every cell and system in the body. Breathing more fully and deeply helps you be more aware, more intuitive, calmer, more alert, and more integrated in body, mind, and spirit. It massages the internal organs so that circulation flows freely delivering blood and oxygen to all parts of the body.

Inhale through your nose to filter out particulates and more directly stimulate the brain.

Singing is a great way to increase respiratory capacity. Also pay attention to your posture: Good posture improves lung capacity.

Exercise

Exercise is important, even when you feel tired. Exercises that are invigorating yet not overtaxing, such as brisk walking, are a good place to start. Research at California State University showed that the more steps you take, the more energy you'll have. If you've been sitting, quickly assess how much energy you have at the moment. Then get up and take a brisk walk, even just a short one. You'll notice the difference!

Stretching is an important part of any exercise program to relieve fatigue. Gentle yoga and stretches for your neck, shoulders, and back, where most of us hold chronic stress and tension, can especially help boost energy. That's because tight muscles are one way you react to real or perceived danger and trigger the fight-or-flight response. When this response becomes chronic, it wears you out, making you feel tired. When you ease the tension in your neck, shoulders, and back, you're signaling your body that it's okay to shut off the fight-or-flight reaction, and as a result, you'll have more energy.

When you have to sit for any length of time, try twirling a pen or pencil in your fingers, or squeeze a stress ball to release the overall tension in your body. Wiggle your foot or tap your fingers very slowly as you stretch and relax the muscles that are tense.

Practical Tips to Build Energy

Reduce exposure. Try to reduce your exposure to chemicals such as those found in cleaning products and personal hygiene products. Clean with more natural products, like white vinegar and baking soda.

Have your water tested for contaminants. If necessary, consider getting a water purifier or using bottled water, preferably bottled in glass.

Avoid overexertion, overwork, and overly processed food.

Employ a good massage therapist. Massage relieves stress and improves circulation and lymphatic drainage.

Have regular times for going to bed and waking up. If you take naps, take them at a regular intervals. Try to establish a rhythm.

Get good sleep. See chapter 14 for help with that.

Set goals. Set a few specific goals for each day and write them down the night before.

Set your schedule. Schedule the most difficult tasks during the time of day when your energy is highest.

Put some color into your life. Reds, bright pinks, and orange tones, whether worn or used in decor, help perk up your energy. During the day, let the sunshine in!

Use music to set the tone for your energy level. When you have to accomplish tasks, play upbeat music. Faster beats can help you get motivated for tasks such as cleaning the house. Slower beats calm the spirit and promote relaxation.

Use water. When showering, end with a brief round of cold water to strengthen the nervous system (you can enhance this by using an invigorating, all-natural peppermint soap). Several times a day, try spraying your face with some cool water that has been lightly scented with peppermint essential oil (20 drops essential oil to 8 ounces water).

Keep your brain engaged. Use your downtime to read more than watching TV. Or choose media that is consciousness elevating.

Write it down. If your troubles are wearing you down, getting your problems out of your mind and onto a piece of paper makes you feel lighter. Brainstorm possible solutions. Talk to someone supportive.

Pray, meditate, and keep those positive affirmations coming. Offer every day for the highest good.

Take the time to rest deeply. Sometimes what you really need is a nap.

Take time to do healthy things for yourself every day!

16
Chronic Pain

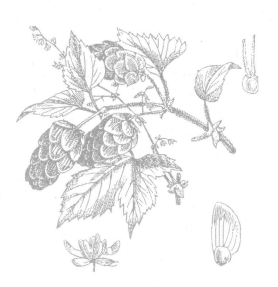

Pain is Nature's way of giving us clues to our body's ailments so that we can do something about them. But that doesn't mean it's easy to deal with. Chronic pain, especially, can be difficult to manage, mentally and emotionally.

Some key elements to consider in the management of pain are contributing factors like sleep, nutrition, and hormonal balance, as well as the underlying cause of the pain. Natural remedies can provide relief from mild to moderate pain and make way for healing. Many forms of holistic medicine consider pain to be a manifestation of stagnant energy, so some remedies focus on moving energy. If your pain does not abate, however, it's important to see your health care practitioner.

What Causes Pain?

Pain is often due to inflammation, which is a protective function that prevents bacteria, toxins, and foreign material at the site of an injury from spreading. When tissues are injured, they release chemicals like histamine that irritate the nerves. Histamine begins the inflammatory process by dilating blood vessels, which increases their permeability so the healing can begin. Kinins are proteins in blood that also dilate blood vessels and increase their permeability, attracting white blood cells to the inflamed site.

COX-1 is an enzyme present in our tissues on a regular basis and produces prostaglandins that help regulate normal body functions. COX-2 is an enzyme not normally present in the body. It is produced only at sites of inflammation, where it catalyses the prostaglandin production that increases inflammation.

Pain messages travel up via nerves to the the spinal cord and from there up to the thalamus (base of the brain). One way that the brain responds to pain is by producing endorphins, which have a morphine-like effect. After this crossing, the pain message then travels to the brain's cerebral cortex.

Many pain-relieving natural remedies target the COX enzymes as a means of inhibiting the production of prostaglandins. Others work to reduce histamine levels or boost endorphin production, among other actions. Some work to raise serotonin levels because low levels of this neurotransmitter increase levels of substance P, a peptide that binds to pain receptors in the brain and spinal cord and directly produces pain.

Nutritional Therapy

Some particularly beneficial foods for someone suffering from pain are those that can reduce inflammation, including brown rice, oats, black-eyed peas, broccoli, cauliflower, cherries, flaxseed, grapes, olive oil, pineapple, sesame seeds, and winter squashes, as well as rosemary, ginger, sage, and turmeric.

Also consider gluten-free grains (millet, black rice, buckwheat, and quinoa), poultry, and raw dairy products; they are good sources of the amino acid tryptophan, which encourages production of serotonin.

Cayenne and other hot peppers stimulate endorphin production. Cayenne also contains capsaicin, a compound that can be applied topically in a prepared cream to deplete the chemicals that transmit pain signals. Strawberries contain natural salicylates, making them cooling and anti-inflammatory. Raw string beans have long been considered a therapeutic food for arthritis for their ability to eliminate uric acid, which can contribute to joint pain. Celery seed also helps eliminate uric acid in the body.

Eat Tart Cherries

Research at the Oregon Health and Science University showed that tart cherry juice has the highest anti-inflammatory content of any food and can help people with osteoarthritis manage their condition better. Cherries contain antioxidants called anthocyanins, which give them their red color and help reduce inflammation. In a study of twenty women aged forty to seventy who had osteoarthritis, the researchers found that drinking tart cherry juice twice daily for three weeks helped reduce inflammation markers.

You can eat tart cherries fresh, dried, or frozen to receive benefits, or drink tart cherry juice twice daily for three weeks, or take a supplement.

Eat Fish

Many types of fish, especially cod, halibut, tuna, flounder, striped bass, salmon, and herring, help relieve pain because they contains a neuro-toxin that works to block the neurological transmission of pain signals to the muscles.

In addition, research published in the journal *Surgical Neurology* in 2006 showed that the omega-3 fatty acids found in fish oil reduce the inflammatory response and, as a result, pain, with no significant side effects.

Sip This

Green tea contains polyphenols, a type of antioxidant that cools the pain and inflammation of rheumatoid arthritis. Research at the University of Michigan Health System in 2007 showed that this compound may inhibit the production of molecules that cause the destruction of cartilage and bone. Drink four cups of green tea a day, or take a supplement of the polyphenol epigallocatechin gallate (EGCG).

Skip This!

Avoid food allergens, which, as we've learned, definitely contribute to inflammation and thus pain. Foods that are potentiators of pain for many people include yeasts, processed meats (hot dogs, bologna, etc.), aged cheese, MSG, and alcohol because they can overstimulate the nervous system and contribute to inflammation. If you have arthritis, you might consider minimizing your consumption of members the nightshade family, such as tomatoes, potatoes, eggplant, and bell peppers. Nightshades contain solanine, which is inflammatory for some and can contribute to arthritis flare-ups.

Supplements for Well-Being

Vitamins B_1, B_6, B_{12}, and calcium can raise your pain threshold. Vitamins C and E are necessary for the production of endorphins. Magnesium can relax muscle spasms; omega-3 fatty acids reduce inflammation and inhibit prostaglandin production.

Vitamin D is also helpful in managing pain. A study published in the medical journal *Pain Medicine* in 2009 showed a link between not enough vitamin D and the amount of narcotic medications needed by chronic pain patients. Researchers at the Mayo Clinic found that those who had low levels of vitamin D needed nearly twice as much medication as those who had normal levels. Your health care practitioner can check your vitamin D levels, as low levels can contribute to fibromyalgia and bone and joint pain. If you are deficient, your practitioner may recommend that you take a vitamin D supplement for natural pain relief.

Bromelain, an enzyme that comes from pineapples, reduces levels of inflammatory prostaglandins. Research shows that bromelain and quercetin work better together.

!

Cure Caution

Bromelain and quercetin are contraindicated for anyone who is pregnant or who has a bleeding disorder or uncontrolled blood pressure.

DL-phenylalanine (DLPA) is made from the essential amino acid phenylalanine. Phenylalanine inhibits enkephalinase, an enzyme that breaks down enkephalins and endorphins, so that the naturally occurring endorphins can survive longer. DLPA helps relieve chronic pain yet does not block the nerve transmission of short-term acute pain. In other words, if you touch a hot stove, you will still know it immediately and quickly move yourself away. Most people obtain pain relief within one to four weeks when using DLPA. Some people who suffer from chronic pain are able to use it for a couple of weeks and then go off it for the next two weeks, yet have pain-relieving benefits that last all month long.

!

Cure Caution

Although DLPA is considered very safe, it should not be used with MAOIs, during pregnancy, or by anyone with phenylketonuria.

Digestive enzyme supplementation is not only helpful in digesting foods, but also for reducing inflammation and easing pain.

Glucosamine helps repair and/or preserve cartilage tissue and also enhances hyaluronic acid, the compound that lubricates and cushions joints. Glucosamine sulphate and chondroitin taken together reduce inflammation, help repair traumatized tissue, and ease pain in the joints. They're effective for moderate knee osteoarthritis. Methylsulfonylmethane (MSM) is sometimes included in glucosamine and chondroitin supplements; it helps promote tissue repair in the body by providing sulfur.

Good to Know!

Dimethyl sulfoxide (DMSO) is a controversial substance, but some have found it helpful for pain. DMSO is actually a solvent by-product from the paper-making industry. It has been prescribed for pain in Russia since 1971. DMSO passes through the tissue, relieves pain, reduces swelling, is a muscle relaxant, has bacteriostatic properties, increases circulation, is analgesic, and can help soften scar tissue. Negative side effects include garlic breath, irritated skin, and blurry vision. Best bet? Try other, safer natural remedies.

You can also take a magnesium glycinate supplement for chronic pain.

Mother Nature's News

There are more than a hundred types of neuropathy, meaning damage, disease, or dysfunction of nerves that causes, among other things, sharp, burning, or shooting pain. It is often associated with issues such as diabetes, hypothyroidism, infection (such as shingles), pinched nerves, injury, and chemotherapy or radiation.

Research published in the medical journal *Drugs in R&D* in 2002 showed that acetyl-L-carnitine is helpful in easing diabetic neuropathy. Alpha-lipoic acid can help with diabetic neuropathy as well, reducing pain and slowing nerve damage, along with improving insulin sensitivity.

Healing Herbs

Many of the herbs that help pain are classified as anesthetics, which numb existing pain either locally or generally; analgesics, which help allay pain when used internally; or anodynes, which are sedating and help keep pain from being perceived by the brain.

- **Cannabis:** Cannabinoids function as signaling agents that calm the nerves of the spine and are also helpful in reducing inflammation.

- **Cayenne:** Stimulates endorphin production. Helpful for arthritis, headache, migraine, pain, and shingles. Topically, it blocks transmission of substance P, which transports pain messages to the brain. A study published in the *Journal of Rheumatology* in 1992 showed that capsaicin (the key ingredient in cayenne pepper) relieves the tenderness and pain of osteoarthritis. You can buy capsaicin cream at your health food store.

- **Chamomile:** A nervine and sedative. A good herb for people who complain about everything. Helpful for migraine, neuralgia, pain, stress, and ulcers.

- **Cloves:** Applied topically to numb pain, such as toothaches. Also helpful for stomachache. Analgesic and anesthetic.

- **Corydalis:** Helps relieve pain from traumatic injury. One of its alkaloids, tetrahydropalmatine, appears to block dopamine receptors in the nervous system. Used for backache, dysmenorrhea, headache, and rheumatism.

- **Cramp bark:** Analgesic, anti-inflammatory, antispasmodic, nervine, and sedative. Used for postpartum pain, rheumatism, and spasms of the legs and lower back. Found in liniments for arthritic joints, sore muscles, and back pain.

- **Feverfew:** Inhibits certain prostaglandins and prevents blood platelet aggregation. Used on a regular basis to prevent migraines.

● **Frankincense:** Inhibits the COX enzyme pathway, thereby reducing inflammatory prostaglandins. Used topically to relieve joint pain. Often found in liniments and salves for sports injuries and arthritis pain. Analgesic, antispasmodic, and nervine.

Mother Nature's News

Ginger contains powerful phenolic compounds and antioxidants such as shogaols, zingerone, and gingerols, which can help reduce pain and inflammation. A review published in the *Journal of Medicinal Food* showed that ginger, like NSAIDs, inhibits the COX enzymes that cause inflammation.

A study conducted at the Miami Veterans Affairs Medical Center and the University of Miami in 2001 showed that a highly purified and standardized ginger extract was effective in reducing the symptoms of knee osteoarthritis.

Ginger compresses can be very comforting for painful conditions. Just dip a clean washcloth into a cup of hot (not scalding) ginger tea and apply to the aching joint. Cover with a dry cloth to help hold in the heat. Replace as needed. You can also use topical creams that contain ginger to ease pain and inflammation and reduce stiffness.

● **Hops:** Sedative to the parasympathetic nervous system. Helps ease headache, insomnia, pain, restlessness, stomachache, and stress. Muscle relaxant, nervine, sedative, and soporific.

● **Kava kava:** Both a skeletal and muscle relaxant as well as a central nervous system depressant. Helps anxiety, cramps, depression, dysmenorrhea, insomnia, neuralgia, pain, and rheumatism. Analgesic, antispasmodic, sedative, and tonic.

❧ **Nettle:** When applied topically, the stinging part of the nettle draws blood to a joint, relieving pain and inflammation. If you're feeling brave, strike an inflamed joint with a fresh cutting from a nettle plant to relieve the pain. But an easier way is to use nettle is to take it as a supplement. Capsules can cause stomach upset, so drink it as a tea.

❧ **Passionflower:** Slows the breakdown of serotonin and norepinephrine. For headache, insomnia, muscle spasms, neuralgia, shingles, and stress. Anti-inflammatory, antispasmodic, nervine, and sedative.

❧ **Saint John's wort:** For nerve and spinal pain. Helps heal damaged nerves when used internally and topically. Used for dysmenorrhea, neuralgia, and rheumatism. Anti-inflammatory, antispasmodic, nervine, sedative, and vulnerary.

❧ **Skullcap:** Sedates the brain and spinal column. Encourages endorphin production. Helpful for arthritis, headache, neuralgia, rheumatism, and spasms. Nervine and sedative.

❧ **Turmeric:** Contains two natural compounds, curcumin and curcuminoids, that decrease inflammation naturally. A study in the medical journal *Arthritis and Rheumatism* in 2006 showed that turmeric may be effective in helping to relieve symptoms of rheumatoid arthritis.

❧ **Valerian:** A smooth muscle and skeletal relaxant as well as central nervous system depressant. Used for headache, migraine, neuralgia, shingles, stress, and trauma. Nervine and sedative. Warming.

❧ **Vervain:** Helps dysmenorrhea, migraine, neuralgia, stress, and general pain. Contains verbenalin, a tranquilizing glucoside. Anti-inflammatory, antispasmodic, nervine, sedative, vasoconstrictor, and vulnerary.

🍃 **White willow:** Contains salicin. Inhibits prostaglandin production. Used for arthritis, backache, headache, joint inflammation, migraine, rheumatism, and general pain. Analgesic, anti-inflammatory, antirheumatic, and tonic. Cooling.

🍃 **Wild lettuce:** Used for general pain and restlessness. Believed to inhibit the spinal column's referral of pain. Analgesic and sedative.

🍃 **Wood betony:** Helps headache, migraine, neuralgia, pain, and stress. Analgesic, antispasmodic, cerebral tonic, circulatory stimulant, nervine, sedative, and vulnerary.

Treatments that can be used topically to reduce pain include castor oil packs, charcoal poultices, hot ginger tea compresses, salt packs (heat salt in a pan and put into a cotton pillowcase), and even cold mashed tofu. Mustard foot baths are an old-time remedy to draw the blood away from an injured area, thus relieving pain.

Homeopathy

Homeopathic remedies that may be helpful for relieving pain include the following:

🍃 **Apis:** For hot, burning pain with swelling in the joints, aggravated by heat, but improved by cold.

🍃 **Arnica:** For pain and swelling from sudden trauma.

🍃 **Belladonna:** For red, hot, swollen joints with pain that comes on suddenly, worsened by touch and motion, but relieved by heat.

🍃 **Bryonia:** For pain activated by movement. For severe pain that is improved by heat and lying still.

🍃 **Rhus tox:** For acute arthritis pain in joints that feel better after movement but have sensitivity to cold and damp.

🍃 **Ruta:** For pain at the site of an old injury, worsened by cold and motion.

Topricin, a homeopathic cream, provides soothing relief for many different types of mild to moderate pain.

Aromatherapy

Wintergreen essential oil contains salicin, a pain-relieving compound that is effective when included in salves and liniments, available at many herbal and natural food stores. Citrus oils like lemon and orange are calming and anti-inflammatory when inhaled.

Tea tree essential oil from the leaves of the *Melaleuca alternifolia* tree is helpful when it comes to reducing inflammation. Apply it topically to reduce inflammation.

Other beneficial oils for pain reduction include birch, cajuput, camphor, chamomile, coriander, eucalyptus, fir, frankincense, geranium, ginger, lavender, peppermint, pine, rosemary, tea tree, and wintergreen—which either help to relax the body, brain, and muscles and/or have inflammation reducing properties. Put any of these essential oils in a diffuser to fill the room with soothing scents.

Mind-Body Therapies
and Practices

There are many mind-body practices you can use to support your physical comfort and your mental and emotional relationship with pain. Below are a several suggestions to help prevent, alleviate, and/or cope with pain—see which ones resonate with you.

Acupuncture
Acupuncture also helps stimulate endorphin production. Research in the medical journal *Complementary Therapies in Medicine* (2007)

indicates that acupuncture provides 50 to 80 percent relief to people with acute or chronic pain. From the traditional Chinese medicine point of view, acupuncture is thought to relieve the stagnation of chi, or energy, in the body. To find a practitioner, visit the website of the American Association of Acupuncture and Oriental Medicine.

Yoga

Yoga helps stimulate the production of feel-good endorphins, which can ease the perception and feeling of pain. In fact, according to a review of research between 2010 and 2013 published in the medical *Journal of Evidence-Based Complementary and Alternative Medicine,* practitioners of yoga had less pain and morning stiffness, were able to be more active, and were less stressed and depressed, with a better perspective on life.

Epsom Salt Baths

Epsom salts are high in magnesium, which soothes and relaxes stiff joints and muscles. Soaking in a warm bath to which you have added 1 pound (455 g) of Epsom salts and five to ten drops of a pain-relieving essential oil will release toxins and relieve pain.

Cold and Heat

Throbbing pain, or an injury that hurts too much to touch, like a banged nose or finger, is best relieved by a cold application, such as an ice pack or cool compress. Sharp pain, on the other hand, is often best remedied by heat, such as a hot water bottle or hot compress. Hot tea, made with pain-relieving herbs, makes an excellent warm compress.

Write It Down

Some people find it helpful to write about their experience with pain in a journal. This may even help you find clues about how to manage pain, such as finding that pain is lessened on the days when you take a walk.

Progressive Relaxation

Progressive relaxation eases pain by triggering the relaxation response. See pages 19–21 for more details.

Practical Tips for Soothing Pain and Discomfort

Practice deep, slow breathing. Visualize inhaling healing light and exhaling the pain out of your body.

Incorporate the color blue. The color blue is considered anti-inflammatory—exposure to blue light, visualizing breathing in the color blue, or simply wearing blue might help ease pain and create a state of calm.

Engage and release. Practice tightening the area around where the pain is centered and then releasing. This can help alleviate the pain.

Have a witness. Often people tolerate pain better if they have friends watching them.

Give yourself a reward. Another thing that can help us tolerate pain is knowing there's a reward at the other end of it!

Draw it out. You can use art to describe your pain by drawing or painting it. Is it like a biting dog or like burning flames? In your mind's eye, gently muzzle the dog or pour water on the fire. Next, draw images that soothe pain and visualize them to find relief.

Try hypnosis and/or magnet therapy. Both therapies can be effective in the treatment of pain.

Most importantly, be kind and gentle with yourself.

17
Grief

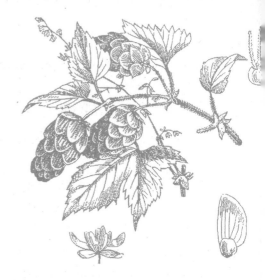

It has been said that "what soap is for the body, tears are for the soul." An essential part of living more harmoniously and happily is learning how to deal with and accept loss: how to let go, recover, and ultimately move on. Grief is a necessary part of our lives. It helps us appreciate what is important and teaches us to be present in the moment, rather than taking all the people and experiences in our lives for granted. But the road from loss to healing and life afterward can be bumpy. These natural remedies can help.

The Effect of Grief on the Body

When you are grieving, your heart rate, blood pressure, hydrochloric acid production, and adrenaline levels rise. You might experience a sensation of numbness, pain along the breastbone, sinus congestion, and broken spasmodic breathing, where you sob easily.

Chronic grief can be a contributing factor in heart disease and arteriosclerosis. It also can lead to a weakened immune system.

Grief

The Traditional Chinese Medicine Perspective

In traditional Chinese medicine (TCM), the metal element, associated with the lungs and large intestines, is connected to the emotion of grief.

Sadness is said to cause a depletion of chi, chronic fatigue, and suscep-
tibility to lung problems.

According to TCM, there are four forms of sorrow:

- Grievious sorrow, which may cause you to break out into loud
  tears
- Mournful sorrow, where you cry quietly, shedding many tears
- Depressive sorrow, where you may not shed tears but show sorrow
  in your face
- Angry sorrow, where you may want to cry but lack tears and
  are unable to make a sound—sorrow embodies anger, and anger
  embodies sorrow

Nutritional Therapy

Foods that can support us during times of grief include green and
orange foods, such as violet leaf, dandelion, kale, collards, carrots, sweet
potatoes, and winter squashes, as they support the lungs and large intestines, which can become more vulnerable when we are grief stricken.
Celery helps comfort the pangs of a broken heart. Pungent spices, such
as clove, coriander, and ginger, can help clear lung stagnation.

Supplements for Well-Being

Craving carbohydrates during periods of grief may be the body's
attempt to elevate serotonin levels. Instead, try the supplement
5-HTP, which helps your body make its own serotonin. GABA can
help relieve cravings, including not just cravings for particular foods
but the desire to have a person who cannot be in your life the way
you would like. The amino acid tyrosine may help elevate moods by
increasing dopamine levels.

Vitamin B complex is a great ally during any time of emotional distress, including grief.

Healing Herbs

Herbs can be a great comforter during times of grief. Calming the nervous sytem through nourishing herbs such as hops, lemon balm, and passionflower can be very beneficial when grieving. Saint John's wort is good to use when you are worn out from sobbing; motherwort is a soothing remedy for grief. For sorrow arising from heartbreak, try this formula, which contains herbs that have long been used in folk medicine for their heartache healing qualities: two parts hawthorn, two parts lemon balm, one part motherwort, and one part violet (also known as "heartsease," for good reason).

Homeopathy

Homeopathic remedies that can be helpful for easing grief include the following:

- **Causticum:** May be of benefit if you cry frequently or are experiencing forgetfulness and mental dullness.

- **Ignatia:** For grief, loss, and hysteria, or if you sigh and can't sleep. You may be nervous and shake. You strongly identify with the person lost and feel you cannot exist without them. Use for disappointment in love or death.

- **Natrum muriaticum:** When you dwell on the past, hold grudges, and reject sympathy. For death and loss of a loved one. When you have not been the same since your loss and are becoming withdrawn, and not living life to the fullest.

- **Pulsatilla:** When you are sad, yielding, indecisive, and weepy. You need to be with other people. Use for anxiety following bad news. For women who can't leave a bad relationship.

Flower Essences

Some flower essences that are helpful include the following:

- **Bleeding Heart:** For grief related to the loss of or separation from a love. Helps foster peace and detachment.

- **Borage:** Use when you are discouraged during times of grief. Helps lift your spirits and gives you courage.

- **Hawthorn:** Gives protection during periods of intense grief and stress.

- **Honeysuckle:** Use when you have made no steps toward recovery even months after the loss of a loved one. You are living in the past.

- **Mustard:** For deep gloom that comes on strong, then suddenly leaves. You may cry without knowing why.

- **Pear:** For extreme grief or emergency situations that throw you off balance.

- **Star of Bethlehem:** For great physical shock and trauma, such as rape, injury, robbery, and accidents. It can also be used when you are having a difficult time coping with death of a pet or loved one. Dr. Edward Bach called this essence "the comforter and soother of pains and sorrows."

Aromatherapy

Soaking in the bathtub can be a good place to let the tears flow. Add any of the following essential oils, all of which are dispellers of grief.

Cedarwood	Marjoram
Clary sage	Neroli
Cypress	Orange
Fir	Patchouli

Frankincense	Rose
Geranium	Rosemary
Ginger	Rosewood
Grapefruit	Sage
Helichrysum	Sandalwood
Hyssop	Spikenard
Lavender	Tangerine
Jasmine	Ylang-ylang

Lemon balm essential oil is a good choice for heartbreak over a love relationship.

When you're done bathing, let the water drain out while you are still in the tub, and visualize your sorrow and sadness going down the drain and being healed by the earth. Afterward, massage diluted essential oil (8 ounces sunflower oil with 30 drops essential oil) over your heart and lungs. Or use the oils in a diffuser, or simply take up to ten deep inhalations directly from the bottle.

Mind-Body Therapies and Practices

Grief can be held in our bodies, our minds, and our hearts. The following are various methods for processing and releasing grief and taking the next steps toward healing.

Good to Know!

The loving support of friends can be a great blessing. When a friend is grieving, "venture, validate, and volunteer": Venture to ask your friend how they are doing. Validate what they are saying; acknowledge their suffering. Then volunteer to help in practical ways, like taking them out to eat, babysitting, giving them a ride, and so on.

Get It Out/Let It Go

It is healthier to express grief than to suppress it. The force of grief is contractive, and expressing it and crying helps clear repression, thus purifying us.

Good to Know!

After crying, asthma, hives, and muscular tension may disappear; blood pressure, pulse rate, and body temperature may lower; and more synchronized brain wave patterns may occur.

Crying releases oxytocin and endorphins, helping clear not just the psyche but also the body and promoting a feeling of calm and relief from pain in the aftermath. If the tears won't come and you feel they might help heal your grief, there is a technique that can help.

☛ Letting Go: How to Trigger Tears of Release

- *First, create a safe space where you will not be disturbed. If others might hear you, give them advance notice to allow you your process without intervention.*
- *Hold on to something like a big teddy bear or a body pillow.*
- *Place one hand on your collarbone. Breathe, pulling air into your chest only as far as your hand. Begin to breathe more rapidly. Make a sound. Hear the feelings in your voice, and go ahead and sound like a crying baby.*
- *Give yourself the space to feel the sadness. Think about what is causing it and let the tears flow.*
- *Accept the reality that the worst has happened. Gently lean into the pain. Stay with it. You'll find that it's not endless.*

Groan It Out

Groaning is also a method you can use to help dissipate sadness and pain. While groaning, think of the reasons for your suffering. When you exhale, visualize sorrow being exhaled from your being.

Let the Sun Shine

You can also release grief by standing facing the rising sun and letting its rays beam on your heart. Visualize the sun healing your grief while you breathe deeply, and the sorrow leaving your heart with each exhalation.

Closure Rituals

Sometimes things end so that we have an opportunity to evolve. Whether grief is due to death of a person, the end of a relationship, or some other loss, you may want to have a closing ritual.

Create an altar by placing a photo of your departed, a sprig of rosemary (for remembrance), and a calming blue candle in a bowl filled with sand or dirt. Anoint the candle with a fragrance that reminds you of your lost one, and etch the lost one's name into the candle.

Light the candle with a prayer of thanks for the lessons you learned in your relationship with the lost one, and as it burns down and out, reflect or write in your journal about the relationship. You can even play a song that reminds you of your lost one.

You might also consider a ritual of writing a letter to get all of your feelings out and burning it in the fireplace, making a toast to a departed loved one, or lighting candles on important dates such as a lost one's birthday.

Write It Out

When going through grief such as divorce, loss of a relationship or job, and the like make a list of one hundred reasons why this life change might be positive or leave you better off than before. At first the task may be difficult, maybe you will only be able to come up with a few reasons, such as having more time to yourself and not having to XYZ. But over time the list may grow, maybe it will even grow to over one hundred reasons. Recognizing the silver lining can be a powerful healing technique.

Here's another method to write out loss:

☛ Writing About Loss

If you are grieving a death or loss of love, it can be very therapeutic to write about it:

1. Start with when you met or your earliest memories, what your feelings, impressions, and expectations.
2. Write out a few of the most memorable moments and events together.
3. Write about how you benefited each another.
4. Make a list of what you have learned from this person or relationship.
5. Write down what you miss about your lost one and perhaps even what bothered you about them.
6. Give your writing a title, make it a story in the book of your life.

Practical Tips for Healing from Grief

Take care of yourself. As you recover, get plenty of rest. Enjoy massages, if possible. Connect with nature and take walks.

Practice deep, slow breathing. Use your breath to cleanse emotions of grief.

Exercise. Use movement to raise dopamine levels.

Surround yourself with love. Call or have over a few of your best friends or closest family and allow them to cheer you up. Seek out those who want to see you happy. The loving support of friends and family members can be a blessing.

Clean up and clear out your house. Use feng shui to make it harmonious. Burn some sage or artemisia to clear away toxic emotions. It helps to have order in your life when you feel out of control.

Find a grief support group.

Travel. When you feel better, and if you can, consider traveling to someplace new. Travel can help the heart and give you new perspectives.

Wear and visualize violet. This color can help you heal from grief.

Wear rose quartz. Sleep with it in your hand and your dreams may have a healing effect upon your heart.

Turn your energy toward something new. Develop talents. Work on personal growth. Take a class. Read self-help books. Learn a new language.

Pray. Ask for spiritual guidance.

Time is a great healer. You will heal, and it helps to make a conscious decision to do so. Remember that setbacks are part of the process. You may feel that you have healed and then have a bad day where the pain of loss is as intense as ever. This is normal, and a sign that healing is happening. You are letting go of the past to make room for something new!

18
Trauma

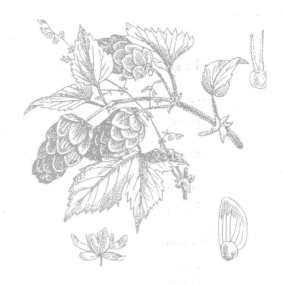

Recovering from trauma, like recovering from grief, is a process that takes time. Trauma can be experienced not just physically but also psychologically, and its effects can be stored in the body and psyche for years afterward.

Trauma can make you feel unsafe in your own body and with others. You may be unable to let go of the anxiety associated with the experience, remaining overwhelmed and terrified. Panic, rage, repetitive destructive behaviors, emotional shutdown, pain, and insomnia may follow traumatic episodes. Nightmares, obsessive memories and thoughts, and a state of hyperalertness can linger.

In this way, trauma becomes an energy locked in the brain and body, exerting a force that can contribute to mental and emotional issues like anxiety, anger, fear, and depression. If you are unable to acknowledge and process that trauma, it can continue to negatively affect your life and relationships.

Positive Support

Having the support of family and friends can be a great ally in healing trauma. If you are the one in the role of offering support, thank the person who is experiencing trauma for trusting you with their feelings. Offer encouragement, such as "I'm here for you, I care, I'm glad you told me." Avoid correcting or analyzing. Don't tell them they should simply get over it; avoid saying, for example, things like "You're fine now" or "Put it behind you." For the person who has experienced trauma, expressing feelings of grief, anger, and hurt may be difficult but can help them release stored emotions and move on. Validate their experience: "*Of course* you feel traumatized." But refrain from painting them as a victim: "Oh, you poor thing."

Keep in mind that if you are a victim of familial trauma—meaning physical, sexual, or emotional abuse in your family—other family members may not understand your point of view or support your recovery because it challenges the status quo and long held assumptions.

As in all cases of trauma, a therapist trained in trauma and support groups can provide support and understanding. For childhood trauma, *Complex PTSD: From Surviving to Thriving* by therapist Pete Walker is an invaluable resource in helping trauma victims understand what happened and how to move forward in a positive direction. Adult Survivors of Child Abuse (ascasupport.org) and Adult Children of Alchoholics and Dysfunctional Families (adultchildren.org) are two organizations that provide resources and host meetings that can help with trauma recovery.

Nutritional Therapy

After a traumatic experience, eat warm, nourishing, comforting foods, like soups. Or ask a friend to make up your favorite dish.

Supplements for Well-Being

An antioxidant supplement can help support healing by helping the body acclimate and repair. Try 7-keto-DHEA to help relieve moods and symptoms associated with post-traumatic stress.

Skip This!

Avoid caffeine, sugar, and other stimulants, which will stress your already frayed nervous system.

Healing Herbs

Soothe the aftereffects of trauma with basil, ginseng, hops, oatstraw, motherwort, raspberry leaf tea, Saint John's wort, skullcap, schisandra berries, and eleuthero. All are nerve-nourishing tonics that can help you heal.

Chinese Patent Medicine

Try the Chinese patent medicine formula called Ding Xin Wan, or Calm Heart Pill, for post-traumatic stress, bad fright, or severe shock to the emotional body.

Homeopathy

Homeopathic arnica is usually the first remedy given after a traumatic event and is good for both physical and emotional trauma as well as trauma in labor and shock.

Aurum metallicum (gold) is good for depression resulting from personal trauma, feelings of anger that surface and are then suppressed, and deep despair and feelings of worthlessness. It helps bring light to those who feel as if a black cloud sits over the future and is a classic remedy for suicidal thoughts.

Flower Essences

Flower essences are gentle, effective remedies for helping to heal the emotional body. After a trauma, the mind and body often store the impact and flower essences provide a safe, noninvasive way to cope with difficult life situations and transform them so we can move into a more balanced state.

Rescue Remedy is the Bach Flower Remedy for panic, shock, grief, despair, and other crises. Take two drops under the tongue to help you find your center again.

Other flower essences to consider for trauma include the following:

🖉 **Hibiscus:** For women who have been sexually traumatized.

🖉 **Mariposa Lily:** Helps alleviate trauma from sexual abuse as a child.

🖉 **Star of Bethlehem:** For great physical shock and trauma, such as rape, injury, robbery, and accidents.

Aromatherapy

Lavender essential oil is calming and relaxing, while rose essential oils help soothe emotional traumas. Take up to deep ten inhalations from the bottle. Or take an aromatherapy bath, using 1 pound of epsom salt and seven drops of lavender or rose essential oil.

Mind-Body Therapies and Practices

When working on healing any condition, it is helpful to incorporate several modalities. T'ai chi and qigong are both practices that can help unlock stored emotions. Gentle self-massage or the gentle tapping of the emotional freedom technique (see page 223) can help you reconnect to your body. Some have found saunas and sweat lodges to be helpful in detoxing and purifying from stressful emotions. Others turn to prayer and calling on a higher power for help with healing. Therapy and even psychedelic therapy can be invaluable in uncovering and relieving the after-effects of trauma.

Certainly not all of these suggestions will be on your current to do list, but finding several that resonate and giving them a try may bring about great things. The self-love and self-exploration involved can help you direct your own healing energy, along with the help of others. (A great source for more exercises on overcoming trauma is Peter A. Levine's *Waking the Tiger.*)

Acupressure
Apply pressure to the point two-thirds of the way from the upper lip to the nose. This point, known as governing vessel 26, helps calm the mind and restore focus after an intense situation.

Meditation and Breathing

Try the practice of breathing in love, breathing out hurt feelings, stressors, or worries.

Take a meditative shower: Take a long, slow shower, directing the spray on various regions of your body—head to feet, front to back—being sure to include every part. Use a pulsing showerhead to help overcome the numbness sometimes associated with trauma. Be present with each part of the body, reminding yourself, for example, "This is my chest, I welcome you back." Use whatever water temperature you find comfortable.

Green Therapy

Surround yourself with the healing color of green, which is in the center of the rainbow, calming the physical and emotional center, the heart. Consider a healthy shade of green clothes, bedding, or foods and have green growing plants in your midst.

Write It Out

Help heal your wounds by writing about your feelings, getting them out of you and onto paper. Once you've done this, you might give your writing to a trusted friend to read, and then discuss it with them.

Above all, be patient and gentle with yourself throughout the healing process.

!

Cure Caution

Don't try to go it alone! Professional counseling and medication can help you recover, even if the trauma occurred years ago. Honesty, awareness, communication, and commitment are essential for healing.

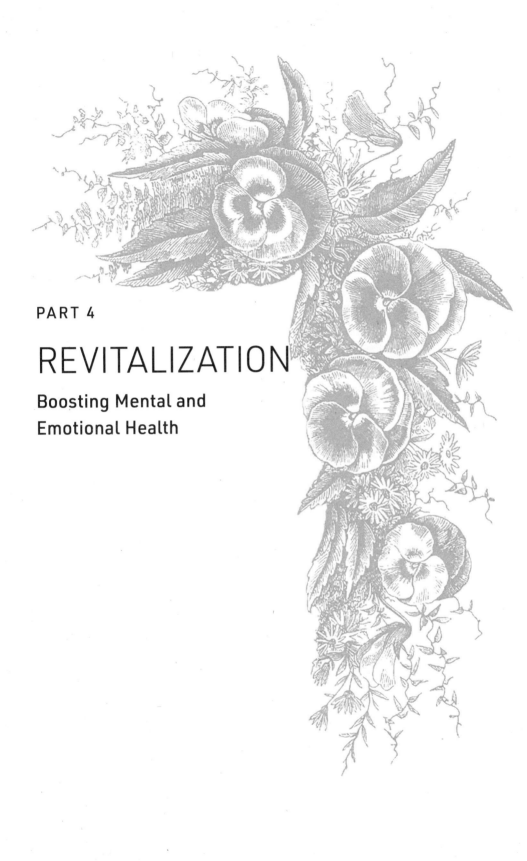

PART 4

REVITALIZATION

Boosting Mental and
Emotional Health

19
Enhancing Cognition and Memory

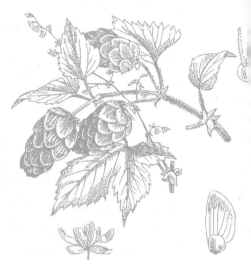

No matter how closely you examine the water, glucose, and electrolyte salts in the human brain, you can't find the point where these molecules became conscious.

DEEPAK CHOPRA

Even though the brain makes up only about 2 percent of our total body weight, it requires about 20 percent of the body's total oxygen intake. The brain of a newborn human baby already weighs one-fourth of its adult weight and can grow one milligram a minute! By age four, the brain has grown to 90 percent of its adult weight, yet the rest of the body is only 20 percent complete in size.

The brain is an amazing organ, but, if you can't remember where you left your keys or your phone—you're not alone. Nutritional deficiencies, foods and behaviors that cause inflammation, aging, and even conditions like hypothyroidism and Lyme disease can affect our ability to think clearly and to remember important things. They can even sometimes lead to chronic diseases like Alzheimer's and Parkinson's. The good news? You can improve the way your brain functions by choosing a better diet for your brain, along with using helpful herbs, supplements, and other natural remedies.

Good to Know!

Brains will sprout new connections between cells to meet demands as long as our environment challenges or stimulates them. Whenever you learn new things, more links are added between neurons. The saying "use it or you lose it" applies to mind and body! The more you know, the more you can know. You may want to check out some of the brain training programs now available, like BrainHQ.

Nutritional Therapy

Foods full of trans and saturated fats contain omega-6 fatty acids, and these encourage the production of inflammatory chemicals called prostaglandins in the body, resulting in free radical damage to the brain and leading to conditions such as Alzheimer's, Parkinson's disease, ADHD, and depression.

Unfortunately, most of us don't get the antioxidants we need to combat oxidative damage.

Foods that are said to best enhance mental alertness are green leafy vegetables (which are rich in chlorophyll, which helps the body better utilize oxygen), coffee, flax seeds, walnuts, cauliflower, chia seeds, blueberries (high in antioxidants), hemp seeds, and cold saltwater fatty fish like salmon, cod, sardines, herring, and mackerel (rich in omega-3 fatty acids).

Omega-3 essential fatty acids are important for brain health because the brain is 60 percent fat. The omega-3 fatty acids known as DHA (docosahexaenoic acid), which is the most abundant fat in the brain, and EPA (eicosapentaenoic acid) improve the health of the cells of your central nervous system and provide structural support so neurons can communicate with each other.

Low DHA levels have been linked to memory loss and Alzheimer's disease, and the older you get, the more you need it. A study published in the medical journal *Alzheimer's and Dementia* in 2010 showed that degenerative conditions like these can be prevented and even reversed with DHA. Elderly volunteers who had memory problems showed improvement after taking 900 mg of DHA for twenty-four weeks. Other research has shown that DHA supports cognitive function in other ways, too, like improving verbal fluency.

If you don't like the taste of fish, get your DHA and EPA in a high-quality fish oil supplement. You may also want to try taking krill oil, which, because of its molecular composition, is absorbed much more effectively than fish oil. Plant-based alpha-linolenic acid, an omega-3 fatty acid from flaxseed, walnut, and hemp seed oil that is converted in the liver into DHA and EPA, is also helpful as an adjunct, but go with fish oil first.

In addition to the foods mentioned above, the following foods can make a difference in brain health by improving mental function, clarity, and memory.

Coconut and its oil. Your brain is fueled by glucose converted by insulin into energy. If you don't have enough glucose, your brain just doesn't function as well. Coconut oil can help. That's because the ketones in the body that help convert fat (as opposed to glucose) into energy come from medium-chain triglycerides (MCTs) found in coconut oil. In fact, coconut oil contains a whopping 66 percent MCTs. Start with 1 teaspoon a day with food and gradually build up to 1 tablespoon (14 g) daily for maximum benefit.

Green tea. Contains catechins, potent antioxidants with powerful anti-inflammatory properties that prevent the kind of damage to nerve cells that is characteristic of such conditions as Alzheimer's and Parkinson's diseases and inhibits COX-2 inflammation.

Nuts. Almonds contain healthful fatty acids like those found in olive oil, with plenty of monounsaturated fat. They also contain 10 IU of the antioxidant vitamin E (alpha-tocopherol) per ounce and are good sources of nutrients such as magnesium, copper, calcium, and riboflavin. Walnuts are a good source of the omega-3 fatty acids that nourish the brain.

Purple and red foods. When you eat blueberries, dark cherries, pomegranates, black grapes, and beets, you tap the power of anthocyanins, strong antioxidants that protect blood vessels. A study in the *American Journal of Clinical Nutrition* (2005) showed that the phytochemicals such as the anthocyanins in blueberries may also enhance signaling between nerve cells. Compounds in blueberries may also make nerve cell receptors more effective in binding with the brain's chemical messengers.

Dark green veggies. These greens contain magnesium, which lowers levels of C-reactive protein (CRP), a blood marker of inflammation. Their antioxidant properties help protect the central nervous system from the damage caused by oxidation. They also improve memory.

Dark chocolate. This treat is high in antioxidants. Choose organic dark chocolate because it is free from pesticides. Compared to milk chocolate, it is also lower in sugar, which promotes inflammation in the body.

Sesame seeds. Antioxidants work to protect the fats that make up the walls of our cells. Studies show that black sesame seeds are even more effective than white sesame seeds in protecting cells against free radical damage.

Turmeric. Research shows that turmeric could be an effective enhancer of an enzyme that protects the brain against oxidative conditions like Alzheimer's disease. It's also well known as for its anti-inflammatory properties.

Mother Nature's News

Quercetin is an antioxidant that helps prevent cell and tissue damage from oxidation. Good sources of quercetin include apples, berries, plums, and onions.

Easy Brain-Boosting Recipes

Try these quick and yummy brain boosting recipes.

Brainiac Smoothie

Consume colorful nutrient dense foods in one delicious drink to reduce inflammation and provide excellent brain nutrients like antioxidants and magnesium!

Makes 1 serving

- 2 cups water
- ¼ cup cacao powder
- ¼ cup blueberries
- ½ banana, sliced
- 1 tablespoon almond butter
- 1 tablespoon maple syrup
- 1 teaspoon ground turmeric

Blend and enjoy.

Breakfast of Champions

This recipe is great when you're on the road or when fresh produce is unavailable. It is high in omega-3 fatty acids, needed for brain health.

Makes 2 servings

- ¼ cup mixture of chopped figs
- ¼ cup sunflower or pumpkin seeds
- ¼ cup whole chia seeds
- 1 cup water

The night before, soak the figs in ½ cup of the water. In a separate bowl, soak the seeds in the remaining ½ cup water. In the morning, drain and rinse the seeds. Add to the rehydrated fruit, and stir well. Enjoy the soaked seeds and fruit mixture as a delicious fiber-filled, brain nourishing way to start the day.

Magic Muse

This snack satisfies sweets cravings and includes foods that improve energy and clear thinking.

Makes 1 serving

   ¼ cup cup raw cacao nibs

   ¼ cup fresh or frozen blueberries

   1 tablespoon raw tahini

   1 tablespoon raw sunflower seeds

   1 teaspoon goji berries

   2 tablepoons maple syrup

   1 tablespoon spring water

Mix together and enjoy.

Super-Greens Salad

One meal a day should include greens as they are high in chlorophyll, which helps the body better utilize oxygen, and they promote many things including clarity of thought.

Makes 2 to 4 servings

   1 bunch kale, young dandelion greens, or collard greens, washed and chopped fine

   2 tablespoons lemon juice

   2 tablespoons olive oil

   ½ teaspoon Celtic sea salt

   ½ teaspoon chili powder

   1 teaspoon nutritional yeast

   1 teaspoon spirulina powder

Toss everything together. Then firmly massage the seasonings into the greens. Let sit for a few minutes, then enjoy.

☙ 10-Second Quick Treat

This easy snack, high in protein and minerals, is a quick energy enhancer. Stuff a pitted date with some almond butter or a Brazil nut.

Supplements for Well-Being

Look to B vitamins first. That's because the entire B complex acts as lubricants for cellular function, and a deficiency can lead to memory loss and impaired cognition. Vitamin B_1 helps the brain transform nutrients from protein and glucose. It can help with mental fatigue as well as memory loss and confusion. A vitamin B_2 deficiency can lead to impaired brain development in the young and behaviorproblems.

Why Vitamin B_{12} Is So Important

Vitamin B_{12} is an essential nutrient in myelin, the fatty sheath that surrounds the nervous system. Low levels can contribute to memory loss. Vitamin B_{12} also helps brings oxygen to the brain cells and reduces inflammation. Highest sources of B_{12} are liver, blue-green algae like chlorella, and brewer's yeast.

Fogginess and problems with memory are two of the top warning signs that you have vitamin B_{12} deficiency, and this is indicative of its importance for your brain health. In fact, a Finnish study published in *Neurology* in 2010 found that if you consume foods rich in B_{12}, you can slash your risk of Alzheimer's later in life.

Good to Know!

Memory loss can be caused by hypothyroidism, hormonal changes, anemia, chronic Lyme disease, and a vitamin B_{12}

deficiency. If you are concerned about your memory, ask your health care practitioner for complete blood tests to get the whole picture.

———————

More Brain-Boosting Nutrients

Other nutrients that support brain health include the following:

- **Beta-carotene and vitamin A:** Help get more oxygen to the brain and help prevent fatigue.

- **Boron:** Helps promote mental alertness.

- **Calcium and magnesium:** Needed for proper brain function. Without magnesium we may be more prone to confusion, lethargy, and depression.

- **Choline:** Increases the brain's rate of metabolism and the metabolism of fats.

- **Coenzyme Q_{10}:** An antioxidant that decreases in our brains as we age.

- **Folate:** Necessary for the production of RNA and DNA, which is essential for memory, learning, and growth in children and for memory in adults.

- **Iron:** Helps make neurotransmitters and DNA.

- **Lecithin:** Used in Europe to treat senility. It also helps in fat metabolism. In healthy people, lecithin accounts for a large component of the brain.

- **Phosphatidylserine:** A phospholipid that can improve memory and cognitive capabilities.

- **Potassium:** Needed to maintain normal levels of neurotransmitters.

◈ **Vitamin C:** A lack of vitamin C can lead to hypersensitivity, fatigue, and depression. Vitamin C is also an antioxidant, protecting delicate nerve cells. Note: Vitamins C and E work synergistically to protect against dementia.

◈ **Vitamin E:** Helps protect the brain from free radical damage and in turn delays the onset of dementia. Elders from Okinawa known for their longevity eat superfoods like sweet potatoes and other foods that are high in vitamin E, like nuts, seeds, olives, vegetable oils, avocados, wheat germ, whole grains, and leafy green vegetables. If you don't get enough vitamin E from your diet, supplements can help. Note: If you take blood-thinning medication, it's very important to check with your doctor before taking any vitamin E supplementation.

Why Your Brain Needs Amino Acids

Amino acid therapy can really improve your mental capacity to enjoy the world.

◈ **Acetyl-L-carnitine:** A form of L-carnitine that improves memory by stabilizing cellular membranes, boosting energy production, and making nerve transmission more effective. It stimulates acetylcholine production and absorption by the brain.

◈ **L-cysteine:** A precursor to N-acetylcysteine (NAC), an antioxidant that helps make glutathione. It improves cognitive function and stabilizes neurological deterioration.

◈ **L-glutamine:** Readily crosses the blood-brain barrier and becomes glutamic acid. It serves as brain fuel and as a protective agent.

◈ **L-methionine:** Nourishes brain cells and helps improve cognitive and neurotransmitter function.

◈ **L-phenylalanine:** Works as a neurotransmitter and is being found to help improve learning ability, mood, and memory.

- **L-taurine:** An antioxidant and an electronic regulator for nerve cells. It is also a chemical transmitter for the brain.

- **L-tyrosine:** Stimulates the production of dopamine, norepinephrine, and epinephrine, promoting alertness and awareness; it is even mood enhancing and motivating. Low levels of dopamine can contribute to depression, autism, schizophrenia, and hyperactivity.

Good to Know!

Since your gut is your second brain—you even have neurons in your gut that produce feel-good neurotransmitters like serotonin—it's important to keep it healthy by avoiding overuse of processed foods, sugar, and antibiotics. Taking a probiotic supplement can help maintain healthy microflora.

Healing Herbs

These herbs have stood the test of time when it comes to helping improve brain function and have been used by various cultures throughout history to improve mental capacities. You can benefit from them today.

- **Ashwagandha:** Supports the nervous system and in ayurvedic medicine is considered a *medhya rasayana* remedy, "a promoter of memory and learning."

- **Bacopa:** Increases attention span and improves memory, learning, and motor coordination. It enhances the ability to learn new tasks and retain new information. Bacopa has been used in ayurvedic medicine for more 1,500 years to improve cognition and recall.

- **Club Moss:** Huperzine, an alkaloid found in club moss, increases levels of acetylcholine in the brain and enhances memory, focus, and concentration. It has been shown to improve Parkinson's and the cognitive factor in Alzheimer's patients. Note: It may be contra-indicated with cholinergic drugs.

🍃 **Ginger and galangal:** Research conducted at RMG Biosciences in Baltimore, Maryland, showed that an extract of ginger and galangal helps inhibit the manufacture of inflammatory brain chemicals and in turn slows the progression of neurodegenerative disorders such as Alzheimer's, which is the most common form of dementia.

🍃 **Ginkgo:** Helps improve the brain's ability to utilize oxygen and glucose by improving peripheral blood flow. Ginkgo has been found to improve nerve signal transmission and activate ATP (adenosine triphosphate), an organic compound that aids metabolic reactions. Ginkgo helps protect nerve cells from free radical damage. Ginkgo is recommended in treating dementia, memory loss, and senility and promoting recovery from stroke. It is an antioxidant and cerebral tonic.

🍃 **Gotu kola:** Used to treat amnesia, dementia, fatigue, and senility. It has a revitalizing effect on the brain cells and nerves.

🍃 **Reishi mushrooms:** Help promote mental clarity and peacefulness.

Chinese Patent Medicine

The traditional Chinese patent medicine Bu Nao Wan, or Cerebral Tonic Pills, helps with poor memory, inability to concentrate, mental agitation, and fatigue.

Good to Know!

Food allergies, yeast overgrowth, addiction, and nutritional deficiencies can all contribute to cognitive impairment and memory loss. Possible contributing factors for Alzheimer's disease, in particular, include inflammation, blood sugar imbalances, toxicity (such as that from aluminum), vascular disorders, head injury, addiction, obesity, chronic infection, and impaired hearing.

Aromatherapy

Since your nasal cavities are very close to the brain, you can use the power of aromas to easily stimulate mental alertness. Try using basil, bay laurel, eucalyptus, ginger, jasmine, lavender, lemon, lemongrass, lime, orange, peppermint, and rosemary essential oils to boost brain power by exciting the neurons.

Cineole, also known as eucalyptol, a compound found in especially high levels in basil, eucalyptus, ginger, orange, peppermint, and rosemary, has been found to increase blood flow to the brain. Ancient Greek scholars wore laurels of rosemary when taking examinations to enhance their memory and Shakespeare wrote, "There's rosemary, that's for remembrance; pray you, love, remember." The uplifting fragrance of this member of the mint family is said to improve memory and increase concentration.

Consider vanilla, too, which is being investigated for its ability to help people recall childhood memories.

Mind-Body Therapies

Use the practices, modalities, and tips below, choosing those that appeal most to you or that address areas you know you need to focus on. Take action to start building brain power today.

Acupressure
A good place to massage to enhance mental alertness is the SI-13 acupuncture point, which is found by reaching your right hand over your left shoulder and, with your middle finger, pressing into the pointy edge

of the shoulder blade on your upper back. Repeat on the other side. This increases blood flow to the brain stem.

Exercise to Boost Brain Power

Exercise increases the body's intake of oxygen and speeds up nerve impulses between brain cells. It increases circulation, gets rid of stress, and cools inflammation. It also encourages nerve cells to produce proteins, such as neurotrophic factor, that improve brain health and cognitive function. Research published in the *Journal of Applied Physiology* in 2012 showed that exercise improves the function of mitochondria that produce energy, and in turn brain power. Other studies show that one hour of exercise five times a week will help prevent degenerative diseases like Alzheimer's.

Choose forms of exercise that you enjoy so you stick with them. If you love to dance, put on your favorite tunes. If you love the snow, try cross-country skiing. If you love the water, swim. Take a walk and watch the world go by. Aim for thirty minutes three or four times a week. You'll notice the difference!

Mother Nature's News

Research shows that keeping your brain active by doing crossword puzzles, reading books or newspapers, writing for pleasure, crafting or other handwork, and playing board games or cards with friends can help prevent dementia and boost mental functioning.

Meditate and/or Pray

Meditate and pray to both calm and expand your consciousness. Prayer is when we talk to Source or Creator. Meditation is an opportunity to be able to listen to Source or Creator. Ideally, you'll meditate daily in the same place at the same time every day. In the morning, soon after awakening and before eating, works well for many people. Sit quietly with your hands resting on your lap or gently beside you. Breathe softly, in and out. Listen to your internal sounds; simply focus on the breath.

Write It Down

Writing helps sharpen, stimulate, and grow the mind. Here are some ideas of what you could write about:

- ▶ Make a list of one hundred things you would like to accomplish in your life. Read over them and write out your reflections.
- ▶ Make a list of three skills you would like to master and elaborate on why.
- ▶ Write out five things you would like to teach your children.

Practical Tips for Building a Better Brain

Expand your experiences and switch it up. Avoid being stuck in a rut and break habitual patterns. Visit new places. Try new foods. Seek out new experiences. Even just traveling to school or work by new routes inspires different thoughts as different sights flash by. Vary the order in which you do things. Shower in the morning instead of at night. Eat breakfast for dinner.

Pay attention. Sharpen your senses by really focusing. Notice as many details as possible. Experience the world using as many senses as possible. Absentmindedness means that the mind was not present or focusing on the matters at hand. Ram Dass was right: "Be here now."

Try it out. An ancient saying goes, "I hear and I forget. I see and I remember. I do and I understand." When learning new things, do your best to do it yourself.

Keep a pen or pencil handy. Always have something to write with. You never know when you are going to get a great idea.

Be young at heart. Play with toys. Collect children's toys and get them out to share with your friends. Play! Allow yourself to have child-like curiosity. My friend Dr. Timothy Leary used to say, "Adulthood is a terminal disease."

Use your body to strengthen your mind. Use your nondominant hand. Using your nondominant hand to complete simple tasks such as brushing your teeth, buttoning clothes, and eating requires you to use the side of the brain opposite the one you normally use. You can also try using your feet instead of your hands to perform a task like putting clothes in the laundry hamper. Practice good posture. This will allow for better flow of energy throughout the nervous system.

Surround yourself with yellow. Color therapists say that the color yellow is cerebrally stimulating. Highlight important passages that you read in yellow, wear the color, and visualize breathing it in. Consider using yellow in lighting and decor in places where mental work is being done.

Quietly and closely, observe nature. She abounds with beauty and intelligence even in minute detail that can inspire us in a positive way.

Free your mind! Write down details—phone numbers, things to do, and goals—to get them out of your head and into action. Keep a calendar with your appointments, tasks, and other logistical details. Nowadays many use the calendars on their phones, but some of us still prefer having it all on paper. Record flashes of brilliance and words of wisdom. Make lists into meaningful categories.

Practice remembering. When you want to remember something, repeat it aloud to yourself. Visualize it being imprinted upon your brain. When learning something important, with your mind's eye, see yourself registering the information and filing it. Then practice retrieving it and refiling it. Use rhyme associations, like the classic "Thirty days hath *September,* April, June, and *November."* To help remember names, associate each name with a picture. *Eileen* has big blue *eyes.* Visualize *Bob* turning into a *bobcat.* Also, right after being introduced to someone, use their name: "It's nice to meet you, Denise." If you don't quite catch the pronounciation of their name, ask them to spell it for you. Make up mnemonics to improve your memory. To remember your license plate number, for example, create a phrase or sentence using words beginning with each of the letters and numbers. For example, MRU607 might be Musk Rat Universe 6 Oh! 7 (bizarre and whimsical is okay). To remember the planets in their order of distance from the sun, take the first letter from each word: Mary's Violet Eyes Make John Stay Up Nights.

Think positively. You'll do better if you affirm that, for example, "I can pass this exam" rather than "I'll never make it."

Engage your mind. Listen to or read self-help programing. Read challenging literature that offers new insights. Read the classics. Enjoy a genre that you have never before read, such as autobiographies, science fiction, or history. Read a magazine with information that is contrary to your beliefs. Ask questions and get answers, even if you have to look them up yourself. Hang out with intelligent people. Converse with interesting people. Have a conversation with someone who has different views than you do. Have in-depth discussions.

Improve your mind with music. Listen to Mozart. Mozart's music has been shown to improve IQ scores. Chopin, Ravel, and Schubert are said to enhance the stream of consciousness.

Avoid substances that damage the body. Try to minimize engagement with substances such as cigarettes, alcohol, pollutants, artificial sweeteners, and MSG.

Study smart. When taking classes, sit in a different place each time to gain a different perspective and foster alertness. When attending lectures, take notes on key words and phrases. When studying, work in the afternoon or right before you go to sleep for better retention of the material. The ideal amount of time to study is thirty-five minutes. In the last five minutes, review what you studied for the first thirty. If you need to study for longer than thirty-five minutes, take a break in between study sessions.

Spend time each day doing nothing. Give the overworked brain time to rest.

Learn about mudras, mantras, and yantras. Mudras are sacred hand gestures. Mantras are sacred chanting. And yantras are pictures that help awaken the divine within. Practice them. For example, chanting the mantra "Om" helps open blockages in the spinal column as well as stimulating the pituitary and pineal glands.

Sleep with rosemary. Keep a sachet of rosemary in your pillowcase to help you to recall dreams. Before going to sleep, tell yourself that you want to remember dreams. Upon awakening, give yourself a few minutes to reflect on and write down the dreams you had. Having a notepad and pencil by the bed may give you the opportunity to record other important thoughts as well.

Draw on the skills and ideas of your friends and coworkers. Practice the art of brainstorming, where you record many wild thoughts and ideas. This often leads to fruitful concepts.

Break chains of blockage and negative thought with diversion. Go for a walk. Call a friend. Go to a movie.

Practice mental gymnastics. Visualization is one method of mental gymnastics. Einstein supposedly came upon the theory of relativity while visualizing flying along at the speed of light. Play mentally challenging games, like chess or Scrabble. Do puzzles, crosswords, and word jumbles. Double a number for as long as you can (2, 4, 8, 16, 32, 64, . . .). Memorize at least one great poem. Take an ordinary object and think of ten other ways it could be used. A book might be a doorstop, a writing pad, a tool to teach you to walk with erect posture, and so on.

Experiment with mind machines. These stimulate various altered states of consciousness. I have found the ones that work with sound frequencies (through headphones) and a wider light spectrum (using a lamp perceived through closed eyes) to be amazing and versatile, providing states of mind from relaxation to high excitement. Many larger cities have places where you can try the machines in stores and even rent them.

Find the best time of day for you to accomplish tasks. Introverts tend to have their most creative time in the early mornings, while extroverts tend to work better at night.

Keep learning things of value for your entire life. Learn two new vocabulary words a week. Use them in a discussion or email. Learn a new fact daily. Read an entry in an encyclopedia daily. It is easier to absorb information if it's gathered gradually than all at once. Learn new skills: language, instruments, dance, martial arts, capoeira, or drawing. Take a class at a local community college. Listen to podcasts and webinars that teach new skills.

Keep things organized. Get rid of clutter and distractions. Learn about feng shui.

Create art. Sketching, sewing, carving, and other forms of creativity open up neural pathways and can create things of beauty. Make a collage or vision board. Create on paper what you want to bring into your life.

Activate your senses. Try getting dressed with your eyes closed. (Lay out your clothes the night before.) Enjoy a meal in the dark or in silence. Wear earplugs when walking to experience deeper levels of silence. Listen to music while smelling an essential oil.

Envision a situation and ask, "What if?" Come up with an answer.

Above all, keep an open heart and open mind. Be open to the possibilities!

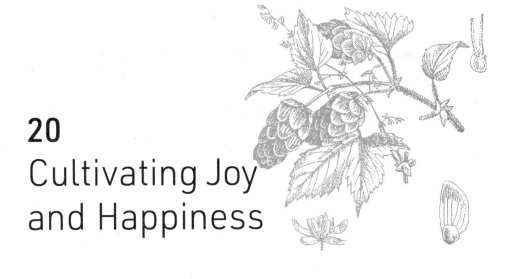

20
Cultivating Joy and Happiness

A merry heart doeth good like a medicine; but a broken spirit drieth the bones.

PROVERBS 17:22

Both happiness and joy contribute to good health, so they are worth learning more about, cultivating, and enjoying. Speaking of joy, this emotion balances the function of the cardiac system and excites the cerebral cortex and the autonomic and sympathetic nervous systems. Joy eases the flow of chi, helping us to relax and feel more harmonious. Happiness increases the activity of the internal organs and rate of digestive secretions.

Nutritional Therapy

According to the principles of traditional Chinese medicine, the heart/ fire system is said to correspond to the emotion of joy. The fire element corresponds to laughter and the spirit, provides energy for circulation, and is often described as "the emperor," ruling all the other organs. An imbalance in the heart or fire element is said to interfere with joy and can manifest as racing heart, speech problems, and sweating easily.

If the fire element is imbalanced in your body, eat more bitter foods such as dandelion leaves and kale and drink reishi mushroom and green tea. Add more colorful, seasonal fresh fruits and vegetables, as well, to make life more joyous by flooding your being with antioxidants and phytonutrients.

Mind-Body Therapies and Practices

Joy isn't something bestowed upon us. It comes from within and, just like all other parts of our wellness, is something we can help create and support in our bodies, minds, hearts, and lives.

Learn about the herb albizia, known as "the happiness herb" and try it as a tea or tincture.

Laughter (Yoga) Is the Best Medicine!

Laughter elevates the levels of feel-good brain chemicals like endorphins that make you feel more positive and happy. Laughter also shakes and caresses the heart, causing it to let go of stored tensions; it dilates blood vessels, improves circulation, increases oxygen intake, and boosts immune health. After a session of laughter, breathing and heart rate slow, blood pressure drops, and muscles relax.

Now there is a yoga practice that encourages jocularity to improve health: laughter yoga. More and more people are practicing laughter yoga each day, and it is now widely used in hospitals to speed healing and to help ease depression in chronically ill patients.

In 2006, Laughter Yoga International commissioned a research project to study laughter yoga's effects on stress levels in IT professionals in Bangalore, India. Half of the group attended seven laughter yoga sessions over an eighteen-day period. The results proved that laughter is the best medicine. The laughter yoga group experienced a significant drop in heart rate, blood pressure, and stress hormones. Laughter yoga also helps promote a positive state of mind. In this study, "glass half full" or positive emotions increased by 17 percent, and "glass half empty" or negative emotions dropped by 27 percent.

If you'd like to join the fun and get healthy, but you have a hard time laughing, zinnia essential oil can help foster lightness, humor, and release of tension and help you delight in life's joy and inner-child wonder.

Write It Out

Journaling can help you set and achieve goals, improve communication skills, reduce stress, and improve confidence and memory. Here are some ideas:

- ▶ Make a list of all the things you love and/or appreciate about yourself.
- ▶ Make a list of the difficulties in your life. Go through the list and see which one of these things you can let go of.
- ▶ Write down what you need to do. Honor your commitments.
- ▶ Make a list of one hundred things you want to accomplish in your life. Put a check by those you achieve. Update the list as you achieve your goals.
- ▶ Make a list of your past successes, awards, and accomplishments.
- ▶ Make a list of ten things you love. Make a list of ten things you are good at. Consider a career based on where some of those things intersect.
- ▶ Make a list of the things you truly are grateful for.
- ▶ Write down all the positive things that happened in a day: seeing a friend, finding something you needed on sale. Strive for at least seven things a day.

Practical Tips for Joy and Happiness

Joyful, happy people are said to live longer. These tips, ideas, and strategies will help you see the sunny side of life more of the time, improving your life, health, and well-being.

Turn your problems over to a Higher Power. Having a spiritual path feeds the soul and keeps you connected to the divine plan of the universe.

Go to the water. When difficulties occur, sit by a river and let go. Learn to go with the flow. Accept and move on. Look for the positive things that can happen from a negative experience.

Get the facts. When you're facing a challenge, getting all the facts can help you accept the situation. Gather data. Ask others to share some insight on the situation.

Process fully, then move on. Instead of brooding over things gone wrong, review the event, then fully experience your feelings for one minute. Afterward, turn your attention to something else. Repeat as often as necessary.

Accept the current reality. Choose to create what you want in life. Take action to create what you want. Focus on the experience you want to have.

Bring more humor into your life. "He who laughs, lasts." Read the comics. Watch comedies. Ask others if they know any good jokes. Learn some yourself!

Associate with positive or inspiring people. Avoid negative influences and people who drag you down.

Share life and joy with loved ones. Spending time with children and having loving relationships can increase your quality of life.

Adopt a pet. People that have pets are likely to live longer and enjoy healthier, happier lives.

Let go of trying to please everyone. Avoid taking things personally. Look for the ways in which you can see yourself in other people, and don't get hung up on the differences.

Communicate your feelings. Those who withdraw are more prone to cancer and suicide. Those who are angry and hostile are more likely candidates for heart attacks. Optimists have fewer chronic diseases.

Pause. Instead of saying yes or no right away, you can say, "I'll think about it."

Help someone in need. Reach out and touch others. Volunteer.

Participate in community activities. They can provide great fun and an opportunity to learn something new as you mingle with others.

Clean out clutter. It contributes to feeling stuck and blocked. Get rid of things that no longer serve.

Rearrange your home. Learn about feng shui as a way to improve every area of your life.

Stop spending money on what you don't need.

Make health a positive priority. This might include good nutrition, meditation, and exercise. Do at least seven healthy things for yourself daily. Have potlucks with friends. Inspire each other to try new foods and eat healthier.

Spend time in nature. This can help you develop inner peace. Get outdoors in full-spectrum light for at least a few minutes each day. Take a walk almost every day.

Create. Creative people tend to be more flexible and enjoy life more. Take up a craft, draw, sculpt, and paint. Making things of beauty improves self-esteem and can help relieve tension.

Keep learning for your whole life.

Plant a garden. It shows belief in the future and brings joy and life lessons daily.

Participate in media consciously. Spend your time reading books that are uplifting and watching shows that have value rather than filling your consciousness with violence and despair.

Recognize the positive already there. Make a list of all your positive attributes. Make a list of all the people in your life you appreciate.

Let go of the past. Every experience in life has taught you something or made you stronger. You can choose to move on from past hurts.

Breathe in joy. Use essential oils that promote feelings of joy, including basil, bergamot, neroli, orange, and rose.

Keep flowers in your home or garden. Use flowers that help calm the spirit and promote joy, including chrysanthemum, jasmine, lotus, narcisuss, orchid, and rose. They may help you lighten up.

Do your best to have a good life. Do something to make the world a little bit better because you were here!

Thank you for beginning your journey to health, happiness and well-being with us. With a little effort, you can make real and lasting changes in your life. Start on the path today by taking the first step!

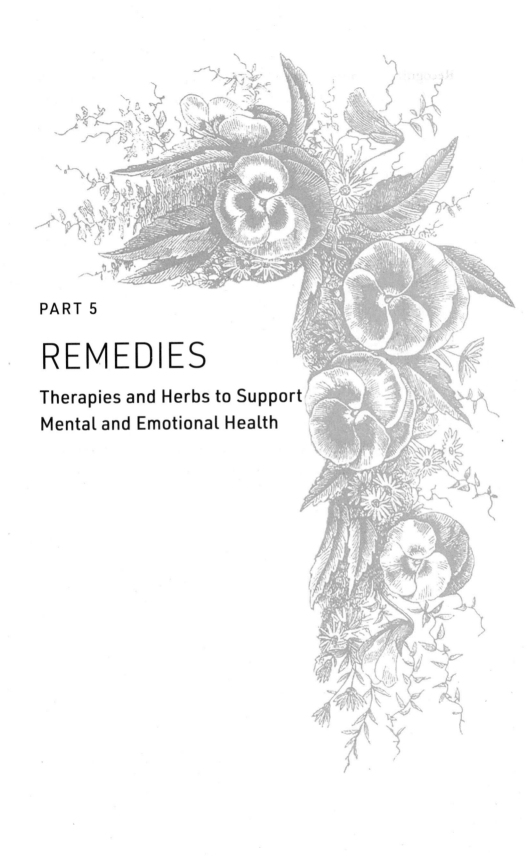

PART 5

REMEDIES

Therapies and Herbs to Support
Mental and Emotional Health

21
Holistic
Therapies:
From A to Z

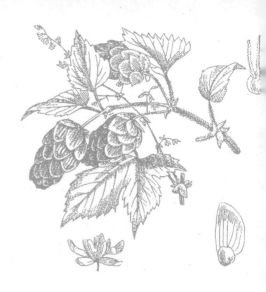

M ore and more people are turning to alternative healing because of its focus on the mind-body connection and the fact that remedies can be tailored to each person's individual needs. In this chapter, we'll explore the wide variety of therapies and practices that can benefit mental and emotional health.

Acupuncture

Traditional Chinese medicine is based on the belief that disease results when chi or the vital life force in the body is disrupted and an imbalance of yin and yang occurs. Yin represents the cold, slow, or passive principle, while yang represents the hot, excited, or active principle.

Chi flows through the body via twelve main meridians, or pathways, and eight secondary meridians. There are more than two thousand acupuncture points on the human body that connect with these meridians. An acupuncturist stimulates these points on by inserting thin metal needles into the skin to relieve blockages to chi. This stimulation also releases pain-killing neurochemicals, such as endorphins and immune system cells, at specific sites in the body.

Acupressure

Acupressure can be seen as a more moderate version of acupuncture that uses finger or tool pressure on the body, rather than piercing the skin. Like acupuncture, acupressure focuses on meridians in the body and releasing any blockages that prevent the healthy flow of energy. Many of the mental and emotional imbalances addressed in this book can be helped by acupressure, as detailed in earlier chapters; simply apply pressure three times for ten seconds each, several times daily, to the specified points.

Aromatherapy

Aromatherapy is the practice of using volatile constituents found in the essential oils of plants to heal the body, mind, and spirit. Essential oils are distilled or pressed from plants and flowers. In nature, the constituents found in essential oils are protective; they help protect plants from fungi, bacteria, and viruses, repel predator insects, and attract beneficial pollinators. In humans, the aromatic constituents of essential oils reach the nose, travel along a neurological pathway, bypassing the blood-brain barrier, and eventually enter the bloodstream, where they stimulate neurotransmitter production and other biochemical reactions.

Note: Genuine aromatherapy utilizes only essential oils derived directly from plants. Be sure you are using pure essential plant oils and not synthetic fragrances. Keep essential oils out of the reach of children and away from light, heat, plastics, and metals. Some oils can stain clothing and damage the finish on furniture.

If you have any questions about using essential oils, please consult a qualified practitioner for guidance. Some essential oils are contraindicated during pregnancy.

How to Enjoy the Aromas

Aromatherapy doesn't have to be complicated. It can be as simple as smelling the flowers! Here are a few simple methods to help you experience the benefits of aromatherapy.

► **Inhaler:** To make an aromatherapy nasal inhaler add five drops of essential oil to ¼ teaspoon Celtic sea salt. Place the ingredients in a small glass vial with a lid. Open and inhale as often as needed.

► **Bath:** Fill your tub with hot water, then add two to eight drops of essential oil and mix well.

► **Room mister:** Mix twenty drops of essential oil with 1 tablespoon of brandy. Pour that mixture into a mister bottle, then add 8 ounces of water. Shake well before using

► **Tissue:** Place several drops of essential oil on a tissue and take deep inhalations.

For External Application

Most essential oils are too strong to use alone and should be diluted in good-quality cold-pressed carrier oil, such as almond, apricot kernel, grape seed, or sunflower oil. Use the following dilutions, depending on the desired total volume:

► 2 drops essential oil per 1 tablespoon carrier oil
► 12 drops essential oil per 1 ounce carrier oil
► 25 drops essential oil per ½ cup of carrier oil

Lavender and tea tree oil are the exceptions; they can be applied neat (undiluted), using no more than five drops at a time.

For any application, if contact with essential oil makes your skin burn, wash with soap and water and then apply vegetable oil directly to the skin.

No person should take essential oils internally except under the guidance of a qualified professional.

Essential Oil Medicine Cabinet

The following essential oils provide a wide variety of benefits including relaxation, mental clarity, energy, and an improved mood, and can be good to have on hand or to start your essential oil collection.

- **Basil:** Helps you find a second wind when you're fatigued.

- **Bay laurel:** Improves concentration and memory and inspires confidence.

- **Bergamot:** Relieves anxiety, depression, and compulsive behavior and encourages the release of pent-up feelngs. A good aid to withdrawal from sugar, food, or alcohol addiction.

- **Cardamom:** Improves concentration; relieves overthinking and worry.

- **Cedarwood:** Promotes strength during times of crisis, boosting confidence and willpower.

- **Chamomile (German):** Eases stress, depression, insomnia, and resentment. It is said to help you let go of fixed expectations and promote a sunnier disposition.

- **Cinnamon:** Stimulates the senses, yet calms the nerves.

- **Clary sage:** Arouses the emotions, eases depression, and helps you feel more grounded in the body. Relieves muscle tension and cramps as well as hormonally related concerns of premenstrual syndrome and menopause.

- **Clove:** Stimulates the thalamus to release enkephalin, a neurochemical that promotes a sense of euphoria and also gives pain relief.

- **Coriander:** A gentle stimulant that helps relieve depression and stress. Has long been used in love potions and as an aphrodisiac.

- **Cypress:** Sedative; helps suppressed feelings surface and be liberated.

- **Eucalyptus:** Decongestant; helps you feel less constricted emotionally; prevents fainting.

- **Fennel:** Stabilizes blood sugar levels; promotes confidence, self-expression, and creativity.

🍂 **Frankincense:** Aids in prayer, meditation, and spiritual self-discipline.

🍂 **Geranium:** Calms anxiety, lifts depression, reduces stress and fatigue, and stimulates sensuality. Helps you feel at ease and aids in resolving passive-aggressive issues.

🍂 **Ginger:** Helps open the heart; aphrodisiac. Improves depression and promotes motivation.

🍂 **Grapefruit:** Helps prevent the urge to overeat as a way to delay dealing with difficult emotions. Cleansing and clarifying; helps clear feelings of frustration, anger, and self-blame.

🍂 **Jasmine:** Fosters feelings of love, confidence, compassion, receptivity, compassion, and physical and emotional well-being. The essential oil has a chemical structure similar to that of human sweat and helps stimulate dopamine production. It relieves stress, moves emotional blocks, calms fear and anxiety, and is mildly euphoric.

🍂 **Juniper:** Helps you break through psychological stagnation and let go of worry and fear of failure.

🍂 **Lavender:** Calming and soothing; relieves anxiety, fear, insomnia, and stress. An excellent bath herb that helps lift the spirits after a difficult day. Eases frustration and irritability; encourages the release of pent-up feelings. Stimulates serotonin production.

🍂 **Lemon:** Antidepressant and emotionally cleansing. Helps relieve irritability and insomnia.

🍂 **Lime:** Has the same uses as lemon. It is uplifting and energizing, helping to dispel worry and clear emotional confusion.

🍂 **Lemon balm:** Calms the spirit; relieves nervous agitation, insomnia, restlessness, and stress. Promotes clarity.

🍂 **Lemongrass:** Antidepressant; promotes mental alertness.

- **Marjoram:** Helps relieve obsessive thinking and obsessive behavior and promotes self-nurturing. Encourages a sense of peace and calms the feeling of neediness.

- **Myrrh:** Relieves worry and promotes focus.

- **Neroli:** Sweet and cooling; relieves anxiety, stress, grief, and depression. Promotes strength and comfort and helps you release repressed emotions.

- **Nutmeg:** Invigorates the brain, calms and strengthens the nerves, and has long been considered an aphrodisiac.

- **Orange:** Anti-inflammatory and sedative; eases tension and frustration, promoting more positive feelings.

- **Patchouli:** Calms anxiety, lifts the spirits, stimulates the nervous system, improves clarity, and attracts sexual love.

- **Peppermint:** Cooling and stimulating, awakening mental activity and relieving fatigue.

- **Petitgrain:** Calms panic and anxiety.

- **Pine:** Promotes confidence and feelings of positivity.

- **Rose:** Associated with physical and spiritual love and is a supreme heart opener. Helps heal grief from emotional trauma; helps you feel happier; relieves anger, depression, jealousy, and relationship conflicts. Good for anyone who feels distanced from their emotional center.

- **Rosemary:** Improves memory, calms anxiety, promotes confidence, and prevents fainting.

- **Sage:** Invokes wisdom and balance, improves memory, lifts depression, and calms fear.

- **Sandalwood:** Can be massaged into the forehead for its calming effects and to enhance meditation. Relieves depression, improves fatigue, and eases coughs.

Good to Know!

Sandalwood trees take at least twenty-five years to grow. In order for the essential oil to be made, the tree needs to be cut down, which is contributing to the decimation of sandalwood trees and the high cost of the oil. Use only sustainably harvested sandalwood products.

- **Spearmint:** Has a lower menthol content and is thus less medicinal and somewhat sweeter and lighter than peppermint.

- **Tea tree:** Stimulates the nerves and helps lift depression.

- **Thyme:** Uplifting and invigorating.

- **Tuberose:** Antidepressant and aphrodisiac; strengthens and evokes the emotions.

- **Vanilla:** Calms and appeases anger and irritability. May stimulate the release of serotonin, causing feelings of arousal and satisfaction.

- **Vetiver:** Uplifting yet calming to an overactive mind.

- **Ylang-ylang:** Calms anger, anxiety, stress, and fear. Relieves depression and frigidity, improves self-esteem, and helps foster a state of peacefulness.

- **Wintergreen:** Analgesic, antiseptic, aromatic, astringent, and stimulant.

Art Therapy

Art therapy is any form of creativity—drawing, painting, sculpting, photography, and so on—that can help you express your emotions and work through anxious feelings. The best art therapy utilizes nontoxic, portable creative endeavors, like sketching, crochet, knitting, or playing an instrument.

To start, you'll work with an art therapist by telling them the issues you are working on, and then you'll be guided through the process of creating as a way to express and resolve how you are feeling. You may find that the process of creating will help you "get out of your own way," as they say, and get a fresh perspective. Art therapy does *not* require any particular artistic skill; it is very effective for anyone working through an emotional or mental health problem, regardless of their artistic ability.

Breath Therapy

Often, we hold our breath without even knowing it or we don't inhale and exhale deeply. But breathing deeply and easily not only nourishes the brain but improves clarity and alertness. When we're stressed, our breathing becomes shallow, but deep breathing boosts the oxygen level in the body, making us feel both relaxed and more energized.

As a general rule, try to breathe in through your nose, which warms the air and helps trap microbes and particles before they reach the lungs. Breathe into your belly rather than only into your chest. As you inhale, you can visualize taking in life force; as you exhale, let go of tensions and toxins. Or visualize that you are the ocean, and your breathing is the waves. Breathe more deeply and fully and do your best to make the exhalation longer than the inhalation.

Conscious breathing exercises can be especially helpful for managing pain, anxiety, stress, and difficult situations. They also immediately place us in the present moment, which is a much calmer, less anxious state of mind. There are several different forms of conscious breathing practices. Try them all.

☞ Deep Relaxation Breath

- *Lie on the floor with a pillow under your knees for support.*
- *Place your palms over your abdomen, with your fingers gently laced just above your navel.*
- *Breathe in for a count of three, pulling air into your belly so your abdomen pushes your fingers toward the ceiling.*
- *Exhale for a count of five as your fingers and abdomen move toward the floor.*
- *Repeat as desired.*

☞ The Complete Breath

- *Lie on the floor with your arms at your sides, palms facing down. Close your eyes.*
- *Slowly inhale through your nose, pulling air down into your belly and then, as your abdomen expands, up into your rib cage and finally your chest.*
- *Hold for a few seconds.*
- *Then breathe out slowly while drawing in your abdomen and relaxing your chest and rib cage.*
- *Next, breathe in slowly as before, but as you pull in air, raise your arms up over your head until the backs of your hands touch the floor.*
- *Stretch and hold for 10 seconds.*
- *As you slowly exhale, bring your arms back over your head to your sides.*
- *Repeat the whole procedure several times.*

☞ Qigong Breathwork

This ancient Chinese practice increases the oxygenation of the blood, tissues, muscles, and organs.

- *To begin, sit or lie down in a comfortable position. Smile to relax your mind and body.*

◆ *Place the tip of your tongue gently against the roof of your mouth and breathe in slowly through your nose.*

◆ *As you exhale, picture any stress in your body or mind transforming into smoke and leaving your body with your breath.*

◆ *Repeat as desired.*

◆ *When you are done, take one more deep breath, then slowly open your eyes and come back to the world around you.*

Words to Breathe By

Worrying about the future and fretting about the past is guaranteed to stress you out. In *The Power of Now*, Eckhart Tolle recommends concentrating on the breath to help move your attention back into the present moment. "All problems are illusions of the mind," he writes. "Focus your attention on the Now and tell me what problem you have at this moment. . . . It is impossible to have a problem when your attention is fully in the Now." You may find that nothing is really wrong, right now.

Instead, breathe, stay in the present moment, *then* act.

Tolle writes, "Wherever you are, be there totally. If you find your here and now intolerable and it makes you unhappy, you have three options: remove yourself from the situation, change it, or accept it totally." When you focus on your breathing, you'll find that much of your stress and fear fades away.

Box Breath

This is a good exercise to do throughout your busy day, and a good reminder to yourself to breathe more deeply and slowly into the belly and chest. As you do this exercise, visualize your breath traveling up your spine as you inhale and down the front of your body as you exhale.

◆ *Sit or stand in a comfortable position.*

◆ *Inhale deeply for a count of five, allowing your chest and belly to expand.*

• Hold for a count of five.

• Inhale a sniff of air, then exhale slowly for a count of five, relaxing your shoulders and pulling your belly inward.

• Hold for a count of five.

• Repeat seven times, or as many as desired.

Color Therapy

Light, as we have seen, can boost hormones, modulate neurotransmitter production, regulate sleep cycles, and influence mood, among other things. Lack of light can contribute to depression, insomnia, and a host of other issues. Color therapy uses the vibrational energies of the different colors of light to nourish and influence our physical and emotional bodies for healing and well-being.

There are specific practices of color therapy, such as Color Puncture, a treatment developed in Germany in which colored beams of light are projected onto various acupuncture points. Even simpler is to consciously take advantage of the healing power of colors in your everyday life. Spending time basking in the golden sun, gazing at the blue sky and the turquoise water, and exploring lush green forests can improve your mood and your mental health. You can also try bringing specific healing colors into your life with the following:

▶ Décor: Pillows, tapestries, lights, and so on

▶ Clothing: Choose your outfits based on the type of energy you think you need

▶ Plants and flowers: To bring in the balancing energy of green, for example, or the cheerfulness of red or the calmness of blue

▶ Visualization: Practice breathing exercises while visualizing your breath as a color, for example, or meditate on the image of a color

▶ Diet: Choose foods by color, which is not only a good way to internalize the energy of that color but also a great way to nourish your body, as naturally colorful foods tend to be nutrient-rich

Let's briefly explore the energies and significances of the various colors.

Red: Red is the most physical of the colors. It vibrates the most slowly and has the longest wavelength. Red is stimulating, hot (yang), and exciting. It is associated with the sympathetic nervous system. It symbolizes vitality, strength, passion, and willpower, and it can help you feel grounded, cheerful, and courageous.

Red can help you overcome inertia, fear, and loneliness and can be used to treat depression, fatigue, low blood pressure, erectile dysfunction, and weakness. Use red when you are feeling run down or when you require a quick burst of energy.

In food, red often indicates the presence of lycopene and vitamin C.

Orange: Orange blends red (physical action) with yellow (wisdom). It symbolizes enthusiasm, outgoingness, optimism, confidence, joyfulness, and courage. It is associated with the sexual center, skin, kidneys, pancreas, spleen, and bronchial tubes.

Orange lifts spirits, fosters humor, and loosens repression. It is a social color and can be helpful as an accent color in spaces where people gather, such as family rooms.

In food, orange often indicates the presence of beta-carotene.

Yellow: Yellow corresponds to the sun and solar plexus. It is warm (yang) and associated with cheerfulness, joy, optimism, practicality, confidence, and illumination. It is also a nerve stimulant and associated with wisdom, knowledge, logic, and the mind.

Yellow can help relieve depression, fear, tension, and mental exhaustion. It can be used to treat issues in the adrenals, gallbladder, liver, muscles, nervous system, pancreas, and stomach. Use it to enhance study, concentration, and communication; it's especially helpful in classrooms, libraries, and study rooms.

In food, yellow often indicates the presence of lutein, magnesium, and vitamin C.

Green: Green combines yellow (wisdom) with blue (spirituality. It corresponds to the wood element, plants, spring, fertility, and hope. It is the color of the heart center, symbolizing healing, balance, compassion, love, transformation, growth, generosity, and peace. It affects the lungs, heart, thymus gland, and immune system.

Green is rejuvenating and anti-inflammatory. It can help calm anger, improve memory, and ease paranoia and nervous exhaustion. Use green for backaches, heart trouble, immune disorders, lupus, allergies, head colds, shock, and trauma and to lower blood pressure. In decorating, green helps create a sense of space and connection to nature.

In food, green often indicates the presence of chlorophyll.

Blue: Blue is a symbol of truth, the color of sky and water. Blue is associated with spirituality, serenity, truth, communication, revelation, trust, and faith. Blue is cool (yin), crisp, clean, and refreshing. It is associated with the throat center. Its effect is calming and instills gentleness and composure.

Blue causes the brain to secrete tranquilizing chemicals. It can be used to counteract violence, restlessness, agitation, hyperactivity, and insomnia and to lower high blood pressure, pulse rate, and brain wave activity. It also calms menstrual cramps, hyperthyroidism, colic, burns, itches, and rashes. Blue is a counterirritant and it is the color of choice for pain and suffering. It makes a beneficial color for a room where rest is the main priority, such as a bedroom or meditation area, but it is not a good color for a social area due to the quietness it evokes.

In food, blue often indicates the presence of flavonoids.

Indigo: Indigo is associated with the third eye (brow), our center of psychic awareness and intuition. It is cool (yin), calming, and antiseptic. It can help balance fear, frustration, and negative emotions and is associated with memory, intuition, and meditation.

Soothing indigo can help you be less aware of pain yet fully conscious. Use it to treat pain, poor motor skills, poor posture, menstrual irregularities, hair loss, and eye and ear disorders. It can be a good choice for bedrooms, meditation areas, and churches.

In food, indigo often indicates the presence of vitamin K.

Violet: Violet has the highest vibration of all the colors and correlates to the crown of the head, the center of cosmic consciousness. With violet, we can be more open to divine power and transcend natural laws. It is cooling (yin), cleansing, antiseptic, soothing, and narcotic. It symbolizes creative imagination and spiritual attainment and corresponds to psychic protection, artistry, and mystery.

Violet can be used to soothe serious mental conditions. It helps normalize hormonal activity, helps curb appetite, and regulates metabolism. Use violet to treat migraines, epilepsy, parasites, dandruff, and baldness and to relieve the side effects of chemotherapy.

In food, violet often indicates the presence of vitamin D.

Craniosacral Therapy

Craniosacral therapy was developed in the 1970s by osteopathic physician and surgeon John E. Upledger to release restrictions in the membranes around the brain and spinal cord so the central nervous system can perform more effectively.

For this therapy, you lie down on a massage or treatment table. Using a very light touch (about the weight of a nickel), the practitioner tests for restrictions in the craniosacral system by monitoring the rhythm of the cerebrospinal fluid and releases any blockages to help the body heal and restore balance. To find a craniosacral practitioner near you and for more information, visit the website of the Upledger Institute.

Emotional Freedom Technique

Emotional freedom technique (EFT) is a psychotherapeutic practice based on the principles of energy medicine, cognitive-behavioral therapy, and neuroscience. The practitioner taps on energy meridian points to release negative emotions from the body's energy field and bring the body back into balance. Tapping helps cleanse the energetic field by distracting habitual thoughts and changing the thought process.

EFT can help calm anxiety and stress, relieve pain, ease depression and grief, reduce addictive cravings and withdrawal symptoms, heal trauma, and release negative emotions.

You can also practice EFT on yourself. Here's how.

☞ EFT at Home

1. *Begin in a standing position with both feet firmly planted on the floor. (You could also do this from a chair, but both feet should still be firmly planted for grounding.)*

2. *Scan your body and note any physical sensations. Do the same for your mental state and note any feelings. Perhaps you have a headache at your temples, or your heart is beating fast, or you have a gnawing feeling in your stomach, or you feel irritation at a friend. Rate your sensations, on a physical and emotional level, on a scale from one to ten— one being the most mild and ten the most intense.*

3. *Next you can do a full body tapping through all of the points below or just choose the location or locations you feel most need attention in that moment. Various schools of thought suggest different lengths of tapping but if you're tapping a single point you could do 7 taps or for tapping various parts of the body you could tap three to five minutes (or longer if you wish). Be sure to tap on both sides of the body where applicable.*
   - *Tap on the center of the top of your head (governing vessel).*
   - *Tap on the inside edge of one eyebrow (yin tang point).*
   - *Tap on the outside edge of each eye (gallbladder meridian).*
   - *Tap on the bone underneath one eye (stomach meridian).*
   - *Tap between your nose and your upper lip (governing vessel).*
   - *Tap between your lower lip and your chin (central vessel).*
   - *Tap on the pinky side of hand (small intestine meridian).*

- *Tap on the beginning of the collarbone, from the midline of the body (kidney meridian).*
- *Tap under the arm (spleen meridian).*
4. *Close your practice by assessing how you feel compared to your initial self-awareness scan and have a drink of water.*

Feng Shui

Feng shui has been used throughout Asia for more than five thousand years to create harmony in life by arranging spaces according to the bagua, or feng shui energy grid. The bagua is represented sometimes as a square, sometimes as an octagon, but in each case it is divided into eight areas around a center point. Each area corresponds to a particular aspect of life: career, new knowledge and wisdom, community, wealth, reputation, children and creativity, helpful people and travel, and health. See the image below.

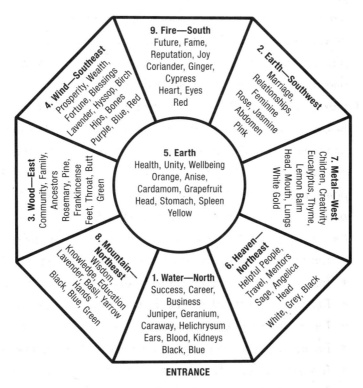

Bagua, or feng shui energy grid
Adapted from a diagram by Rachael Carlevale.

When we arrange our living spaces in alignment with the bagua, we bring success and harmony into every aspect of our lives.

To access the energy of the bagua, our first task is to eliminate clutter. This is because clutter causes confusion and stagnation, leaving us uneasy, stressed, and overwhelmed. So, clear, clean, and declutter and create a living environment of healing, comfort, and beauty as best you can. Start in one room and move on to the next. Once that's done, apply the principles of feng shui in every room, using the main entrance as the key to the grid. Focus on what you'd like to improve. You can find many do-it-yourself guides to feng shui in books and online, or you can seek out a feng shui practitioner in your area.

Flower Essences

Flower essences were discovered by noted homeopath and bacteriologist Edward Bach in England in the 1930s. Flower essences are a diluted "sun tea" of specific wildflowers or tree flowers known for their healing properties that is diluted (similar to homeopathic remedies) and used to balance emotions and encourage healing. Bach Flower Remedies, as they're known, are dispensed over the counter and have no contraindications or side effects. They're nontoxic, nonaddictive, and safe even for infants, the elderly, plants, and animals. All of the Bach flower essences are now also offered in a non-alcohol tincture as well.

The following list provides some brief descriptions for which emotional patterns particular Bach Flower Remedies suggested throughout this book might help. For a full list and further understanding of the thirty-eight Bach flower essences please visit the Bach Original Flower Remedies website.

One can use a single remedy or up to six. Two drops can be placed directly in a cup of water or you can prepare a dropper bottle with two drops from each remedy placed in a clean glass dropper bottle with spring water and a tablespoon of brandy as a preservative—use two drops under the tongue.

Original Bach Flower Remedies

🍃 **Agrimony:** For those who hide their troubles behind a smile. Promotes true cheer from inner joy and self acceptance.

🍃 **Aspen:** For those who feel anxious, fearful, and worried, but not sure why. Enhances inner peace, fearlessness, and sense of security.

🍃 **Cerato:** For those who know what they want to do but doubt their judgment and seek the advice of others. Connects you to inner wisdom and increases self-assurance.

🍃 **Cherry Plum:** For those who feel desperate and like they might lose control. Promotes rational thinking and a calm mind.

🍃 **Chestnut Bud:** For those who continue to make the same mistakes, those who don't learn from the past. Helps you observe your own patterns more objectively and begin to change them.

🍃 **Clematis:** For those who daydream, are ungrounded, are not in their body or the present. Facilitates more interest, presence, and enjoyment in life.

🍃 **Crab Apple:** For those who have a poor self-image, dislike something about themselves, and feel unclean. Promotes self-acceptance despite imperfections.

🍃 **Gentian:** For those who feel discouraged and depressed after a setback. Helps with the realization that doing your best is what counts most.

🍃 **Gorse:** For despair and those who feel hopelessness when things go wrong. Restores a sense of hope and faith even though there may still be problems.

🍃 **Heather:** For self-preoccupation and talkativeness leading to loneliness. Promotes better listening, generosity, and helpfulness to others.

Holly: For those who feel wounded, jealous, spiteful, or vengeful. Enables a more generous heart without making demands.

Honeysuckle: Your mind is on the past rather than the present. Helps one be more present and able to let go of life's regrets and move on.

Hornbeam: For putting things off and feeling tired at the thought of starting work. Promotes inner strength and the ability to face each day.

Impatiens: For impatience and irritation with the slow pace of people or things. Enables more spontaneity, yet with clear decision making.

Larch: For those who expect to fail, lack confidence in their skills, and therefore refrain from trying. Promotes determination, reasonable self-esteem, and more capability.

Mimulus: For fear of illness, death, and accidents. For those who feel shy or anxious about something specific. Fosters quiet courage to surf the vicissitudes of life with more confidence and humor.

Mustard: For those who feel depressed and gloomy and don't know why. Promotes the return of joy and inner peace.

Olive: For those who feel tired after making an effort and continue to struggle despite exhaustion. Restores peace of mind and interest in and joy of life.

Red Chestnut: For anxiety over someone else's safety. For those who are overly concerned for the welfare of others. Enables caring with compassion without anxiety.

Rock Rose: For extreme terror about something, especially after having an accident, trauma, or nightmares. Promotes calm courage and more presence.

- **Rock Water:** For those who drive themselves hard to set an example and are inflexible. Fosters being able to hold high standards with more flexibility.

- **Star of Bethlehem:** For the effects of a shock or grief. Helps neutralize the trauma from either a recent or past incident.

- **Sweet Chestnut:** For despair. For those who feel there is no hope left. Helps liberate one from despair and promotes peace of mind.

- **Walnut:** For big life changes. For those who are unsettled by times of change and who are knocked off course by other's ideas. Helps one stay on one's life course without getting derailed by others. Protects against outside influences that cause anger.

- **White Chestnut:** For persistent unwanted thoughts, preoccupation, insomnia, or nervous worry. Helps the mind become clear and thoughts reasonable.

- **Wild Rose:** For those who lack motivation or can't be bothered. Fosters more engagement and interest in life, work, and the world.

Rescue Remedy is a homeopathic preparation (available in health food stores) made from five flower essences. It can be given in more acute situations such as for trauma, accidents, and emotional distress to help restore calm and bolster confidence. The essences in the mixture are: Star of Bethlehem for shock, Rock Rose for terror and panic, Impatiens for stress and tension, Cherry Plum for despair and fear of losing control, and Clematis for loss of consciousness or feeling "out of it." Two to four drops can be placed under the tongue and held there a minute or so before swallowing. The drops can also be mixed into a small glass of water and sipped. If the person to whom you are administering first aid is unconscious, place the drops on the lips, wrists, back of the neck, or behind the ears.

Herbal Medicine

Did you know that approximately 30 percent of modern drugs have their basis in plant medicine? Pharmaceutical companies routinely send ethnobotanists and pharmacognosists into remote areas of the world to observe what more "primitive" peoples are using in healing. When those researchers bring home traditional medicinal plants, the quest begins for the "active constituent," which very often turns out to be an alkaloid. Some examples of such alkaloids include caffeine, morphine, nicotine, cocaine, quinine, and salicin, many of which are made into strong drugs.

But it's important to remember that a plant is not solely an alkaloid. When constituents are extracted and isolated and turned into drugs, those drugs are missing vital compounds found in the whole plant. Plants are, in fact, powerhouses of biochemical intelligence, containing not just alkaloids but, for example, chlorophyll, essential oils, glycosides, vitamins, minerals, fiber, and other secondary components—many of which increase the plants' effectiveness and help prevent side effects.

Chapter 17 offers profiles of the numerous herbs with amazing benefits for the brain, mental health, and emotional balance.

Dosage Guidelines

Dosages depend in part on which herbs and preparations you're talking about. If you're using a commercial herb product, follow the dosage guidelines on the product packaging, unless you have researched adequately or been guided by a qualified health professional to use less or more than recommended.

If you've made your own tea or tincture, in general, one 8-ounce cup of tea or one dropperful of tincture qualifies as a single dose. For an acute, serious, right-there-in-your-face type of illness, one dose every hour or two would be appropriate except while sleeping—rest is good medicine in its own right.

For a chronic health concern, one dose three or four times daily would be appropriate. Some herbalists recommend pulsing remedies for chronic conditions, which means ten days on, three days off, in a continuing cycle. Pulsing helps the body acclimate and learn to respond even without the herbs. Another pulsing regimen is six days on, one day off, with a three-day break every two or three weeks.

When you are using herbs for therapeutic purposes, continue with the appropriate dosage for at least a week and then evaluate your progress. If your health concern has been remedied, you can stop taking the herb formula on a regular basis. However, you might wish to include some of the herbs you've been using in your diet from time to time as a tonic tune-up.

Special Situations

The dosage guidelines discussed above are generally true for adults. However, dosages may need to be adjusted for different people or different categories of people. For example:

- ► Large people need more than small people.
- ► Women may need less than men.
- ► For the elderly, reduce the dose by one-fourth for those over sixty-five and by one-half for those over seventy.

Homeopathy

Homeopathy is based on the law of similars, or the philosophy that "like cures like." The term *homeopathy* comes from the Greek words *homeo,* meaning "similar," and *pathos,* meaning "suffering or disease," and was developed by Dr. Samuel Hahnemann (1755–1843).

Each homeopathic solution contains an infinitesimal amount of the substance it is made from. You might say it contains a pattern replica of the substance. Exposure to this energetic pattern triggers a powerful healing response from the body. In other words, by stimulating the body's own healing response, a homeopathic remedy encourages the body to heal itself.

Homeopathic remedies can effect amazingly fast-acting and pro-found cures. The degree of success, however, depends on selecting the right remedy for a person's constitution, so although you can diagnose and treat yourself, you may also benefit from consultation with a pro-fessional homeopath to gain insight into the best remedies for your constitution. Note that homeopathy often calls for very small doses of substances that in large doses could be toxic. *Do not confuse homeopathic remedies with herbal remedies.*

Homeopathic remedies come in the form of small pellets, alcohol solutions, or water solutions and are usually safe when taken with con-ventional drugs. Usually, four pellets are placed under the tongue and allowed to dissolve there. It is best to not eat or drink anything for ten minutes before or after taking the remedy. Some homeopaths recommend avoiding coffee, mint, and camphor while using homeopathic remedies.

Contact your health care practitioner if your symptoms do not improve within five days or if you are pregnant or nursing. Keep all homeopathic remedies out of the reach of children.

Homeopathic Medicine Cabinet

Homeopathy is well worth learning about and certainly visiting a skilled homeopath can be helpful but here we have some of the most common remedies that might be used to remedy a wide range of mental, emotional, and neurological concerns. Read through the description for each cure and see which one sounds most like you, then try it. (You do not need to have all of the health concerns or symptoms mentioned in order for a remedy to be the right one for you.)

🍃 **Aconitum napellus (aconite):** Remedy for sudden fright or acute fear. You fear death, darkness, evil, crowds, and even crossing the street. You experience anguish, anxiety, despair, insomnia, restless-ness, and franticness. You wake up frightened with palpitations and are sensitive to light, noise, and touch. You lack appetite. You have anxiety when reminded of a disturbing past.

- **Argentum nitricum (silver nitrate):** For anxiety before an interview or exam. You are impulsive and fear impending events, crowds, and heights. You have panic attacks and diarrhea when anticipating challenging circumstances. You have seizures that occur at night, with menses, or when stressed.

- **Anacardium orientale (cashew):** You have anticipatory anxiety, difficulty concentrating, low self-confidence, and fear of failure and insanity.

- **Arnica montana (arnica flower):** You are experiencing or have experienced shock, trauma (physical and emotional), pain, surgery (before and after), or labor. Arnica is usually the first remedy given after a traumatic event. It aids in reabsorption of fibrin, a blood protein that forms as a result of internal injuries, thereby reducing swelling and bruising.

- **Arsenicum album (white arsenic):** You are fussy, obsessive, overanxious, restless, fault finding, and fearful; you worry about the past and future. Your mind is never at rest, and you toss and turn when sleeping. You want everything to be just right and are always in motion. You fear being alone, losing control, illness, death, incurable diseases, and darkness. You usually have a frail constitution and are cold and thin. You may experience vertigo and memory loss. You may be suspicious and demanding or dislike being in a situation over which you have no control. Arsenicum album is appropriate for anxiety, fearfulness, restlessness, agitation, depression, exhaustion, vomiting, fear of poisoning, burning pain in a lower limb, and extreme thirst. Symptoms are worse after eating and with warmth, and better after midnight and when cool.

- **Aurum metallicum (gold):** You have lost love and feel dull and stupid and even happy at the thought of death. Use for depression resulting from personal trauma, where feelings of anger surface and are then suppressed, or from loss in a business venture, when you feel in deep despair and worthless. Aurum people are often leaders, noble and successful in their fields. When loss or failure occurs, you can feel deeply affected and may turn to prayer. You feel as if a black cloud sits over the future. You feel devalued, sullen, and brooding. You may have been a leader or extremely successful and have substance abuse issues. A classic remedy for suicidal thoughts.

Calcarea carbonica (carbonate of lime): You may be anxious about your health and about catching infections. You fear disease, misfortune, insanity, and loss of reason. You are tired and anxious and perspire easily. You're easily discouraged or methodical. You are breaking down from overwork.

Calcarea ostrearum (calcium carbonate): You feel sluggish, lazy, and apathetic. You have trouble verbalizing, feel old and tired, and often sit around feeling sorry for yourself. You may feel cold, with your feet feeling especially chilled. You may have night sweats or shortness of breath, or you feel confused and depressed.

Capsicum annuum (cayenne): You dwell in the past; you feel homesick, irritable, or depressed, or you want to be somewhere else. An overly emotional person, you may feel threatened by new life situations.

Causticum (lime and potassium bicarbonate): You are depressed due to death of a parent or friend. You feel negative, gloomy, and anxious. You cry frequently and over small things. You feel anxious foreboding that something is about to happen. You may be experiencing forgetfulness and mental dullness. You worry about others rather than yourself. You experience more problems on the right side of your body. Paralysis affects specific parts of your body, such as your face. You are thirsty, and you fear darkness and death.

Chamomilla (chamomile): You are constantly discontented, or you are anxious and impatient. You cry out in sleep.

🍃 **Coffea cruda (coffee):** You have paralyzing anxiety preceding an event such as flying or public speaking. Mental activity causes insomnia. You are excited and nervous.

🍃 **Gelsemium (yellow jasmine):** You are paralyzed with grief following a loss and may tremble. You can't cry. You have mild depression following illness such as the flu. Your anxiety is based on some kind of fear, such as fear of an exam or of public speaking. You're trembling and may freeze up physically and mentally. You are quiet, weak, dull, and apathetic, but not thirsty.

🍃 **Hypericum (Saint John's wort):** You have a nerve injury to areas with lots of nerves, such as fingers, toes, and spine. Or you've had a crushing injury with sharp, shooting pain. Or you have an old injury and nerve pain still bothers you. Or you have pain resulting from dental work.

🍃 **Ignatia (St. Ignatius's bean):** You are disappointed in love. You have suffered a great loss, such as the death of a child, parent, friend, or pet. You feel that you cannot exist without them. You are grieving, with sighing, sobbing, insomnia, and unpredictable behavior. You may alternate between crying and laughing or tend to hold back tears. You have postpartum depression accompanied by hysteria and disappointment. Your anxiety, fear, restlessness, and loud sighs indicate your anguish when you have difficulty expressing your feelings. You get a stomachache or headache after emotional upheaval. Sadness leads to anxiety, depression, hysteria, and anger. You may fear getting fat and rejection. You are obsessive about your weight. You may be nervous and shaking.

🍃 **Kali phosphoricum (potassium phosphate):** You are anxious, overworked, worried, excited, and oversensitive to pain. You may cry easily, scream during sleep, and feel cold frequently. You are prone to dizziness, fainting, laughing fits, and poor memory and suffer from anxiety, gloominess, and shyness. You have nervous exhaustion. You are anxious and exhausted from worrying about relatives. You have weak extremities, fatigue, pain, or prolapse of the eye, with symptoms made worse by exertion. You have may have epilepsy and feel cold after a seizure.

🍃 **Lachesis (lance-headed viper):** Your depression is worse in the morning and during transitions such as menopause. You have outbursts and irrational jealousy. You're domineering, vicious, suspicious, and talkative. You believe you're being conspired against. You need open air and have a wild imagination. You have nighttime anxiety.

🍃 **Lycopodium (club moss):** You suffer from fear, anxiety, and insecurity. You're overly concerned about what people think of you, fear rejection, and think others are being critical of you. You fear animals, aging, change, and loss of position. You are insecure and take out your anger on others. You lack self-confidence about new endeavors. You're indecisive and irritable, but when put on the spot, you excel. You are an intellectual and basically a loner, yet you like to have someone in the house.

🍃 **Mercurius (mercury):** You experience sudden anger with a possible impulse to do violence to yourself or others. You are restless and agitated, you lack concentration, and you have poor memory and rapid speech. You're aggravated by many environmental influences and comfortable in few conditions.

🍃 **Natrum muriaticum (common salt):** You may dwell in the past, reject sympathy, and prefer to be left alone or get violent if someone attempts to comfort you. You may be sad from failed romance, feel anxious about everything, and experience prolonged grief. You are gloomy and overly sensitive to comments. You are tearful, emotional, or irritable yet practical. You suffer from chronic grief, having suffered great unresolved emotional pain, as well as loss of or separation from a loved one. You're easily hurt and hold on to grudges and the past. You dislike going to social events where there will be lots of people. You have fearful dreams or dislike heat, noise, and excitement, which worsens your anxiety. You may appear cool and aloof in order to avoid sharing sorrow, be unable to express anger, and appear overly responsible.

- **Natrum sulphuricum (sodium sulfate):** You've had a head injury and now suffer from depression or seizures.

- **Nitricum acidum (nitric acid):** You feel anxious and depressed. You may have extreme sensitivity to noise and touch. You may have a chronic, painful problem with one of the body's orifices.

- **Nux vomica (poison nut):** You are irritable, critical, and domineering. You can't sleep due to job stress, business loss, overeating, or overindulgences in alcohol. You have anger and possibly a violent temper and destructive impulses. You are fussy and fastidious over small things and dislike being contraindicated. You're hurried and impatient and overemphasize achievement. You're a workaholic or overworked. You're preoccupied with the past, wishing you had dealt differently with a previous experience. You may have numbness in your face, appear to be drunk, and have difficulty in swallowing. Your symptoms worsen with light, noise, and draft.

- **Phosphoricum acidum (phosphoric acid):** You suffer from extreme mental fatigue and burnout. You may respond slowly or not at all to questions. Talking makes you feel weak, and you prefer to be left alone. You're indifferent, silent, and withdrawn due to stress and worry. You may be depressed, lazy, drowsy, and confused and feel like your head is heavy. Overwork can make you predisposed to feeling overwhelmed. You are apathetic toward yourself and food. This remedy can be used for adolescent depression, chronic fatigue, and long-term grief.

🌿 **Phosphorus (phosphorus):** You're fretful and irritable. You laugh hysterically, then cry. You're very sensitive to outside influences. You feel something negative is about to happen. You fear the dark, thunder, ghosts, storms, and solitude. Sleep improves your condition. You may be tall, thin, and excessively sensitive and have an active imagination.

🌿 **Platina (platinum):** You feel superior, arrogant, and prideful. You live on past glories yet lack effectiveness in the present. You are obsessive about your appearance. You may be an egomaniac.

🌿 **Pulsatilla (pasque flower):** Depression alternates with a mild, easygoing manner. You're brokenhearted, weep openly, and yielding; you seek sympathy and may even be clingy. You need to be with other people. Fresh air improves your symptoms. Use Pulsatilla for anxiety following bad news, for women who can't leave a bad relationship, for fear that causes lots of tears and may include fear of dogs, snakes, and insanity.

🌿 **Sepia (ink from the cuttlefish):** You may feel suicidal and miserable over life. Lacking joy, you feel despairing and irritable. You may cry frequently with no desire to work or change. You were once a loving person yet now find life impossible. This worsens as the day progresses. You have an aversion to family and friends. You dread that something might happen. You are indifferent to life and want to be alone. You are disgusted by food and odors, which cause nausea. You are critical of partners, argumentative, and pessimistic. This is a remedy for women who have emotional issues due to hormonal imbalance, like postpartum blues and menstrual-related depression.

🌿 **Silicea (silicon dioxide):** Shy yet strong-willed, you get anxious about exams, public speaking, and interviews, thinking you will lack in your performance. You may feel numb in your fingers, toes, and back. You're easily fatigued and cry easily. You fear the future and failure, though you often succeed. You are melancholy, with difficulty concentrating. You may suffer from nighttime seizures. This remedy is a specific for fear of needles, for those of you who have been putting off acupuncture treatments.

- **Staphysagria (larkspur):** Your ailments are caused by repressed anger. You hold in your temper until you blow up. You are easily offended or sharp-tongued. You have low self-esteem and are unable to express your needs. You may have a hard time sleeping and lie awake wishing you had said or done something different.

- **Sulphur (sulphur):** Ragged and sloppy, you often dwell on religious and philosophical questions. You may be anxious about your soul's salvation and suffer from delusions, yet you are too lazy to help yourself. You're slow and often hungry for cold drinks, sweets, and spices. You may be a know-it-all or someone who is haughty yet philosophical, creative, impractical, or argumentative for the entertainment of it.

Journaling

Writing about your feelings can be a great way to get things out of your consciousness and off your chest. For example, rather than talking repeatedly about a traumatic event, spending hours a day in revisiting a trauma zone, consider writing about the event with every gory detail. You can also include in your journaling what you may have learned from a given event or emotion and how you might move forward. Use what you find to take action!

Massage Therapy

Massage improves circulation, fosters detoxification and lymph drainage, and enhances immune function. Since much of illness and imbalance is stress related, massage improves health by helping you to relax. Not to mention that the act of being touched itself is good for mind, body, and spirit.

Massage therapy can be an excellent method for stress management. Different types of therapy include Swedish massage (most common), aromatherapy massage (with essential oils), hot stone massage (using heated, smooth stones), deep tissue massage (targets deeper levels of muscles and connective tissue), and shiatsu (a type of Japanese bodywork).

Meditation

Millions of people around the planet regularly practice meditation, a mind-body practice that uses certain techniques, such as focused attention (on a word, an object, or the breath, for example), a specific posture, or a neutral attitude toward distracting thoughts and emotions, to foster mindfulness and well-being.

By quieting your thoughts in meditation, you can learn to detach from what is commonly called the "monkey mind," which is your inner dialogue full of judgments and comments about what is going on around you. Practicing meditation will also improve your blood pressure, bolster your immune system, promote a sense of well-being, and reduce stress and anxiety.

There are many wonderful guided meditation programs available. Here's a quick guide to doing it yourself.

☛ Beginner's Meditation

- *Sit or lie down in a comfortable position and close your eyes.*
- *Allow your breath to fall into a natural rhythm.*
- *Settle your attention on your breath. Notice the sensation of your in-breath. Notice the sensation of your out-breath.*
- *When distracting thoughts come, notice them, too, and let them pass. Return your attention to your breath.*

- *Continue focusing on your breath for just a couple of minutes. (Over time, you can increase the length of time for your meditation.)*
- *When you are finished, slowly open your eyes and gently recenter in your day.*

Psychedelic Therapy

Psychedelics are substances that can enlarge the scope of our mind and bring dormant parts of consciousness to the surface. They have been used to aid spiritual practice, explore the self, dissolve the ego, enhance social interactions, increase sensory experiences, and treat disease. They have a low potential for abuse and are rarely associated with dependence.

Today, researchers are exploring the use of psychedelics in enhancing creativity, reducing the incidence of cluster headaches, relieving pain, calming fear of death, and treating post-traumatic stress disorder, depression, and obsessive-compulsive disorder, among other mental, emotional, and neurological imbalances.

Microdosing

Microdosing, which has become popular of late, refers to using a small dosage (about one-tenth what is usually used for a psychedelic effect). The feeling is considered subperceptual but can help calm anxiety and deter cravings for addictive substances. Microdosing can help people become more aware of patterns that contribute to imbalances and facilitate letting go of mental chatter and maintaining a more positive attitude.

Psychedelics activate the brain's serotonin network, which promotes calm and a sense of well-being. They also enhance neuroplasticity—the brain's ability to make new neural connections and maintain flexibility in its processing patterns—which can be key to managing brain injuries and neurological disorders.

On a more metaphysical level, we know that psychedelics give us the opportunity to dive deep into our subconscious, immerse ourselves in our inherent one-ness with the universe, and have deep spiritual epiphanies. Perhaps seeing beyond the mundane, exploring our psyche and the roots of our ailments, and feeling more connected to a divine plan boosts our potential to overcome mental and emotional distress.

Psychedelic substances are more therapeutic than escapist, and they often intensify issues that are already present. When people use psychedelics, it is not uncommon for their past trauma and early childhood experiences to surface. They may initially experience powerful visions and altered states of consciousness. A rising sense of wholeness with people and the universe is a common experience.

Physically, psychedelics may cause dilated pupils, slightly elevated blood pressure and heart rate, numbness, trembling in the extremities, lack of muscle coordination, increased salivation and watering of the eyes, occasional vomiting, elevated temperature, sweating, and goosebumps. Increased sensual perception and visual imagery usually occur. Though using psychedelics carries risks, those risks are usually far less than the risks associated with most addictions.

For more information on using psychedelics, check out the Erowid website or see *Addiction-Free Naturally,* by Brigitte Mars.

Psychotherapy

Finding a qualified therapist can often help resolve complex mental and emotional issues that can't be untangled on your own. The key is to find a therapist who specializes in your area of concern—whether it's anxiety, depression, trauma, addiction, an eating disorder, or something else—and with whom you can build trust and connection. You can find listings for numerous qualified therapists who specialize in different types of counseling on the *Psychology Today* website. Sometimes you need to sample several therapists before you find the right fit, so don't give up if you feel you can benefit from this process. Healing can take a quantum leap forward with the right therapist at your side.

Qigong

The name *qigong* derives from *qi* (or *chi*), "energy," and *gong* (or *kung*), "skill or practice." Qigong originated some five thousand years ago when Chinese scholars studying the workings of the universe concluded that everything is energy, as did Albert Einstein much later. The theory of qigong is that you become sick when energy in your body is out of balance, whether that be too much or not enough. Qigong practice is a form of exercise that helps change the flow of energy in the body, resulting in improved wellness. (You can visit the Qigong Institute website for a directory of qigong teachers, therapists, and classes.)

Reflexology

Reflexology dates as far back as ancient Egypt, India, and China and is the practice of stimulating pressure points in the feet, hands, and ears that correspond to areas in the rest of the body. Reflexology assists the self-healing process by balancing life energy or chi in the body. It is also profoundly relaxing. So, for example, when you rub the point between your index finger and your thumb (L4, or large intestine 4), you treat the pain of migraine headaches.

Sound Healing

Sound healing correlates to using vibration from voice or instruments to tap into energies beyond the physical in order to retune the body, mind, and spirit. You can find practitioners offering sound healing or sound baths, as the practice is sometimes called, via local holistic health clinics. For an at-home version, look for sound healing music online, such as that offered by Jonathan Goldman. You can also try humming, something so simple anyone can do it: Simply take a few deep breaths, then hum up from your mouth, with your lips closed, into your nose. Follow with a short silent break. Humming can reduce stress, improve sleep, lower blood pressure, and improve lymph flow and melatonin production. It also creates new neural pathways, clears the sinuses, and releases endorphins.

Yoga

Millions of people around the world practice yoga, an ancient tradition that began as a spiritual practice in India. By performing poses (asanas), you find health and vitality through increased oxygen intake and the release of endorphins. Yoga also improves flexibility, strength, and muscle tone.

Yoga is a powerful antidote to stress and a way to "be" in the present moment. Yoga postures have a direct effect on health, helping to remove toxins, improve nourishment of the cells of the body, and reduce blood pressure, anxiety, and stress. The practice of yoga also helps you befriend your own body, accepting it as it is. This in turn helps you to accept life on its own terms instead of the way you wish it could be. Without this conflict, life becomes much more peaceful.

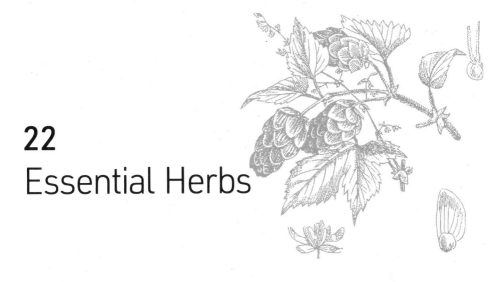

22
Essential Herbs

The essential herbs are listed in alphabetical order for easy searching. On page 287, you will find lists of tea herbs to aid specific conditions and enhance aspects of well-being.

ASHWAGANDHA

Botanical name: *Withania somnifera*
Family: Solanaceae (Nightshade)
Parts used: root (primarily), leaf, berry, seed

Physiological Effects
Adaptogen, analgesic, anti-inflammatory, antioxidant, antispasmodic, hypotensive, nervine, nutritive, rejuvenative, sedative, tonic

Medicinal Uses
Ashwagandha's use has been recorded for at least 3,000 years. It builds chi, helps lower cortisol levels, makes the body more resistant to stress (it even helps prevent stress-releated ulcers), and prevents depletion of vitamin C. It nourishes and calms the mind, decreases anxiety and pain, and promotes sleep, and it has been shown to improve cognitive function in the elderly. Use it for anxiety, bipolar depression, exhaustion, memory loss, mental fatigue, neuroses, overwork, panic attacks, and stress. It is excellent for those in convalescence.

This herb works best when taken over a prolonged period of time. An ayurvedic maxim says that taking ashwagandha for fifteen days imparts strength to the emaciated body, just as rain does to a crop.

Considerations

During pregnancy, use ashwagandha only under the guidance of a health care professional, as there have been some reports of the herb having abortifacient properties. Using this herb in combination with barbiturates can exacerbate their effects. The berries can cause gastrointestinal distress when consumed by children. Do not use the leaf in cases of congestion.

BACOPA

Botanical name: *Bacopa monnieri*
Family: Scrophulariaceae (Figwort)
Part used: aboveground plant

Physiological Effects

Adaptogen, antidepressant, antifungal, anti-inflammatory, antioxidant, antirheumatic, antiseptic, antispasmodic, anxiolytic, bronchial dilator, cardiotonic, carminative, diuretic, immune tonic, laxative, nervine, nervous system tonic, rejuvenative, sedative

Medicinal Uses

In ayurvedic medicine, bacopa is considered *medhya rasayana,* an herb that benefits the mind and spirit, and it has long been used to calm restlessness in children. It is a nourishing brain, nerve, and kidney tonic. It enhances neurotransmitter function, increases production of calming serotonin, and helps protect the synaptic functions of the nerves in the hippocampus, which is considered the seat of memory. It also increases protein synthesis and brain cell activity. It has been found to help chelate heavy metals out of the body.

Bacopa is used in the treatment of ADHD, agitation, Alzheimer's disease, anxiety, asthma, bronchitis, depression, epilepsy, hyperactivity, hypertension, insomnia, irritable bowel, learning disability, memory loss, mental illness, pain, restlessness, and stress.

Considerations

Bacopa is generally regarded as safe, even for children. Not enough is currently known about its use during pregnancy, however, so for now it is best to avoid its use during that time. Take care not to confuse bacopa with gotu kola; both are sometimes called by *brahmi*.

BASIL

Botanical name: *Ocimum* spp., including
O. americanum (American basil),
O. basilicum (sweet basil),
O. citriodorum (lemon basil),
O. gratissimum (tree basil),
O. minimum (bush basil), and
O. tenuiflorum (holy basil)
Family: Lamiaceae (Mint)
Part used: aboveground portion

Physiological Effects

Antidepressant, anti-inflammatory, antioxidant, antiseptic, antispasmodic, carminative, circulatory stimulant, nervine, sedative

Medicinal Uses

Basil stimulates the lungs, warms the body, calms the stomach, and dries dampness. It also inhibits COX-2-related inflammation. It is used in the treatment of anxiety, depression, drug overdose or withdrawal, dysentery, exhaustion, headache, hysteria, nausea, rheumatism, stomachache, and vomiting.

Considerations

Generally regarded as safe.

BLACK COHOSH

Botanical name: *Actaea racemosa*
Family: Ranunculaceae (Buttercup)
Parts used: rhizome, root

Physiological Effects
Anti-inflammatory, antirheumatic, antispasmodic, central nervous system depressant, circulatory stimulant, hypoglycemic, hypotensive, muscle relaxant, sedative, vasodilator

Medicinal Uses
Black cohosh improves circulation and lowers blood pressure. It can be helpful in cases of emotional instability, hysteria, mania, melancholy, moodiness, stress, and anxiety related to menopause. Its potassium and magnesium content contribute to its nerve sedative properties. It has long been considered a remedy for "doom and gloom" depression as well as depression resulting from hormonal conditions arising postpartum, during menopause, or during the menstrual cycle.

Considerations
Avoid black cohosh during pregnancy and while nursing, except under the guidance of a qualified health care practitioner. Avoid also in cases of heart conditions. Excessive use can irritate the nervous system and cause nausea, vomiting, headache, and low blood pressure.

Black cohosh is at risk of becoming endangered in the wild, so instead of wild crafting, consider cultivating your own supplies. When purchasing black cohosh products, be sure they are made only from cultivated stock.

CACAO

Botanical name: *Theobroma cacao*
Family: Malvaceae (Mallow)
Part used: seed

Physiological Effects
Antioxidant, aphrodisiac, cardiotonic, diuretic, nervous system stimulant, nutritive

Medicinal Uses
Cacao increases levels of serotonin and endorphins in the body. It gives a short-term boost in energy. It also contains phenylethylamine, a compound that is naturally occurring in the brain in trace amounts and is released when we are in love, peaking during orgasm. Cacao also contains theobromine, a compound that dilates the coronary artery, increasing blood flow to the heart.

Considerations
In some cases cacao may cause heartburn or an allergic reaction. Since it contains caffeine, it should be used only rarely by pregnant women and can aggravate insomnia, anxiety, irritability, and breast cysts. Cacao also contains oxalic acid, which can inhibit calcium absorption and promote kidney stones.

CALIFORNIA POPPY

Botanical name: *Eschscholzia californica*
Family: Papaveraceae (Poppy)
Part used: aboveground plant

Physiological Effects
Analgesic, anodyne, antispasmodic, hypnotic, nervine, sedative, soporific

Medicinal Uses
Although it does not contain opiates, this poppy is a skeletal relaxant that encourages restoration of the nervous system, and it is nonaddictive. The Cahuilla Native American tribe once used the plant as a sedative for babies. Today, it is used in the treatment of anxiety, bedwetting (due to stress), headache, insomnia, overexcitability, pain, restlessness, stress, and toothache.

Considerations
Avoid in cases of depression. Excessive use can cause one to feel hung over in the morning.

CANNABIS

Botanical name: *Cannabis sativa*
Family: Cannabaceae (Cannabis)
Parts used: bud (flowering top of female plant), resin, leaf, seed

Physiological Effects
Bud, resin, leaf: analgesic, anesthetic, anticonvulsant, antidepressant, antiemetic, anti-inflammatory, antispasmodic, aphrodisiac (but can also be anaphrodisiac, depending on dosage and circumstance), appetite stimulant, bronchial dilator, cataleptic, cerebral sedative, euphoric, hallucinogen, hypnotic, hypotensive, vasodilator
   Seed: demulcent, laxative, nutritive, yin tonic

Medicinal Uses
Cannabis, often called marijuana (among many other names!), contain cannabinoids. The human body contains an endogenous cannabinoid (endocannabinoid) system, implying that we evolved in interaction with this plant. Specialized cannabinoid receptor sites are found throughout the body (including in the bones, brain, nervous system, reproductive organs, spleen, and spinal cord) and help regulate cellular function. The

cannabinoids thus function as signaling agents, helping the body cope with stress, including pain and inflammation.

Cannabis bud's effects can vary in different people, but most noted are the dilation of blood vessels and alveoli sacs in the lungs, resulting in deeper respiration and an increase in heart rate. Low doses tend to promote a sense of relaxation. The bud increases levels of phenylethylamine, a neurotransmitter that makes us feel more in love. The bud is used in the treatment of AIDS, amyotrophic lateral sclerosis (ALS, a.k.a. Lou Gehrig's disease), anorexia, anxiety, appetite loss, asthma, cerebral palsy, chemotherapy nausea, coughs (spasmodic), depression, epilepsy, fibromyalgia, glaucoma, insomnia, menstrual cramps, migraines, multiple sclerosis, muscle spasms, nausea, nervousness in the elderly, nightmares, Parkinson's disease, spastic paralysis, and suicidal thoughts.

Between 1840 and 1900 more than a hundred published medical papers recommended cannabis leaf to aid sleep, calm the nerves, relieve pain and nausea, and stimulate appetite. The leaf is not psychoactive unless processed with heat, such as by being cooked in oil.

Though cannabis is most often smoked to achieve therapeutic effect, it can also be consumed as food, tinctured, encapsulated, or made into a sublingual spray.

In terms of topical applications, marijuana leaves can be used as a poultice or liniment to ease muscle spasms.

Considerations

Smoking marijuana buds may affect some people adversely, possibly inducing paranoia, personality deviations, short-term memory loss, and perceptual distortions. Because of these possible effects and marijuana's sedative properties, try to avoid driving, operating heavy machinery, or other activities that require fast reaction times after taking marijuana.

Smoking in general can be hard on the lungs, and though cannabis buds have been used to treat asthma and bronchitis, smoking them can aggravate those conditions. Marijuana buds can also inhibit testosterone production, cause hypoglycemic states, and lower HCL production.

Dryness in the mouth and eyes is a common side effect. Avoid preparations that rely on a butane inhaler or extracts using solvents like hexane and butane.

CBD is one of the many identified constituents of cannabis. Among other uses, it can be helpful for sleep and anxiety. CBD can be appropriate for those that do not want to get "high" as it can be extracted and used on its own without any significant amount of THC—meaning the mildly psychedelic effect of cannabis is absent.

The seeds are generally regarded as safe.

CATNIP

Botanical name: *Nepeta cataria*
Family: Lamiaceae (Mint)
Part used: leaf

Physiological Effects
Anodyne, antispasmodic, aromatic, emmenagogue, febrifuge, nervine, sedative

Medicinal Uses
Catnip contains nepetalactones, which are both analgesic and sedative, affecting the opioid receptor sites of the body. Catnip moves chi, relaxes the nerves, and calms inflammation. It is an excellent children's herb and will help calm them through the trials of teething, colic, and restlessness. When given for colds and fevers, it helps the patient get the rest they need.

Catnip was entered into the United States Pharmacopoeia from 1842 to 1882 and into the National Formulary from 1916 to 1950. Today, catnip is used to treat anxiety, convulsions, headache, hyperactivity, hysteria, insomnia, menstrual cramps, motion sickness, nervous stomachache, pain, and restlessness.

Considerations
Large doses can be emetic. Smoking it can be hallucinatory. Not recommeneded during pregnancy.

CHAMOMILE

Botanical name: *Matricaria recutita,*
aka *Matricaria chamomilla* (German chamomile)
Family: Asteraceae (daisy) family
Part used: flower

Physiological Effects
Analgesic, anodyne, antifungal, anti-inflammatory, antioxidant, antiseptic, antispasmodic, nervine, sedative, stomachic, tonic

Medicinal Uses
Chamomile is rich in nutrients that support the nerves and muscles, including calcium, magnesium, potassium, and B vitamins. Since the time of ancient Greece, it has been used as a gentle relaxant that tones the nervous system. It moves chi, relaxes the nerves, reduces inflammation, clears toxins, and promotes sleep. As a nerve restorative, it calms anxiety and stress. It's a useful herb for those who are "bothered by almost everything" and has traditionally been used to calm those prone to nightmares. Add chamomile tea to a child's bath before bed to help them sleep peacefully.

Considerations
Some people, especially those who are sensitive to ragweed, may be allergic to chamomile. It can cause contact dermatitis in some individuals. Roman chamomile is more likely to cause an allergic reaction than the German variety. On the other hand, chamomile is sometimes used to treat allergies. Use the herb with caution the first time you try it. Otherwise, chamomile is considered very safe. Avoid therapeutic dosages during pregnancy.

DANDELION

Botanical name: *Taraxacum officinale*
Family: Asteraceae (Daisy)
Part used: root

Physiological Effects

Anodyne, antibacterial, antifungal, anti-inflammatory, antirheumatic, aperient, cholagogue, choleretic, decongestant, deobstruent, depurative, hepatic, hypnotic, laxative, lithotriptic, nutritive, sedative, tonic

Medicinal Uses

Dandelion is one of the planet's most famous and useful weeds. This wonderful plant is a blood purifier that aids in the process of filtering and straining wastes from the bloodstream. It cools heat and clears infection from the body. Dandelion is also used to help clear the body of old emotions, such as anger and fear, that can be stored in the liver and kidneys. The root is used primarily for problems related to the liver and to treat alcoholism, allergies, anorexia, appetite loss, candida, depression, dizziness, fatigue, hangover, headache, hypertension, hypochondria, hypoglycemia, obesity, and premenstrual syndrome.

Considerations

Dandelion is generally regarded as safe, even in large amounts and even during pregnancy. However, as is the case with any plant, there is always a possibility of an allergic reaction. A very few cases have been reported of abdominal discomfort, loose stools, nausea, and heartburn associated with dandelion. The fresh latex of the plant can cause contact dermatitis in some sensitive individuals.

Consult with a qualified health care practitioner prior to using dandelion in cases of obstructed bile duct or gallstones.

ELEUTHERO

Botanical name: *Eleutherococcus senticosus, E. gracilistylus*
Family: Araliaceae (Ginseng)
Parts used: root, root bark, leaf (to a lesser degree)

Physiological Effects

Analgesic, anti-inflammatory, antioxidant, antirheumatic, antispasmodic, blood pressure regulator, hypoglycemic, hypotensive, metabolic regulator, rejuvenative, stomachic, tonic (adrenal, cardiac, chi, immune, nerve, and yang tonic), vasodilator

Medicinal Uses

Eleuthero has been used as medicine in Siberia and China for more than four thousand years. As an ancient Chinese proverb puts it: "Better a handful of eleuthero than a cartload of gold and jewels." In the frigid regions of China, Russia, and Japan, reindeer, a symbol of strength and endurance, consume this plant.

Russian cosmonauts since 1962 have been given rations of eleuthero to help them acclimate to the stresses of being weightless and living in space. Athletes, deep-sea divers, rescue workers, and explorers all use it for support during times of stress. It shares many of the same therapeutic properties as Asian ginseng *(Panax ginseng)*.

Eleuthero helps the body cope with stress and nourishes the adrenals; it is considered an adaptogen. It improves endurance, mood, work performance and productivity. It is used in the treatment of anxiety, alcoholism, exhaustion, chronic fatigue, and weakness.

Considerations

In rare cases, eleuthero may contribute to diarrhea, elevation of blood pressure, and mild blood-platelet antiaggregation properties. Taking eleuthero too close to bedtime may interfere with sleep.

GINGER

Botanical name: *Zingiber officinale*
Family: Zingiberaceae (Ginger)
Part used: rhizome

Physiological Effects
Analgesic, anti-inflammatory, antispasmodic, aphrodisiac, stimulant

Medicinal Uses
Ginger has been found to be even more effective than Dramamine in curbing motion sickness, without causing drowsiness. As a digestive aid, it warms the digestive organs, stimulates digestive secretions, increases the amylase concentration in saliva, and facilitates the digestion of starches and fatty foods.

It also strengthens the tissues of the heart, activates the immune system, prevents blood platelet aggregation and leukotriene formation, and inhibits COX-2-related inflammation and thus prostaglandin production, thereby reducing inflammation and pain. Ginger is used in the treatment of anxiety, depression, fatigue, headache, hypertension, hypothyroidism, indigestion, obesity, and pain.

Topically, ginger can be prepared as a compress and applied over arthritic joints, bunions, sore muscles, and toothaches to relieve pain; over the kidneys to relieve the pain of and assist in the passage of stones; over the chest or back to relieve asthma symptoms; or over the temples to relieve headache.

Considerations
Although ginger can relieve morning sickness, pregnant women should not ingest more than 1 gram daily. Avoid in cases of peptic ulcers, hyperacidity, or other hot, inflammatory conditions. Avoid excessive amounts of ginger in cases of acne, eczema, or herpes.

Ginger may cause adverse reactions when used in combination

with anticoagulant drugs such as warfarin or aspirin; if you are using such medications, seek the advice of a qualified health care practitioner before commencing use of ginger.

GINKGO

Botanical name: *Ginkgo biloba*
Family: Ginkgoaceae (Ginkgo)
Part used: leaf (harvested when it is starting to yellow, then dried)

Physiological Effects

Brain tonic, neuroprotective, rejuvenative

Medicinal Uses

The oldest tree species on the planet, ginkgo was present even when dinosaurs roamed the earth! It has a high resistance to disease, insects, and pollution, which is perhaps one reason why it offers so much protective power to humans too.

Ginkgo has been found to improve nerve signal transmission and activate ATP (adenosine triposphate), an organic compound that aids metabolic reactions. It also helps protect nerve cells from free radical damage. It helps relax blood vessels, improving circulation and the delivery of nutrients, including oxygen and glucose, throughout the body, including the brain. Concentrated ginkgo leaf increases the synthesis of dopamine, norepinephrine, and other neurotransmitters. It may prevent the age-related decline of serotonin production.

Ginkgo can be used in the treatment of Alzheimer's disease, anxiety, dementia, depression, fatigue, memory loss, neuropathy, and pain in the extremities. It can also help in recovery from stroke and brain injury.

Considerations

Side effects from ginkgo are rare. However, large amounts or concentrations have been reported to cause gastrointestinal disturbance, irritability, restlessness, and headache. Ginkgo leaf can negatively affect the blood's ability to clot, so avoid it for at least a week before surgery, in cases of hemophilia, or in concurrence with anticoagulant drugs such as warfarin, aspirin, or MAOIs.

GINSENG

Botanical name: *Panax ginseng* (Asian ginseng),
P. quinquefolium (American ginseng)
Family: Araliaceae (Ginseng)
Part used: root

Physiological Effects
Adaptogen, analgesic, antiallergenic, anti-inflammatory, antioxidant, antispasmodic, chi tonic, digestive, endocrine tonic, hepatoprotective, hypoglycemic, hypotensive, immune tonic, nervine, nutritive, phytoandrogenic, rejuvenative, restorative, stimulant, tonic

Medicinal Uses
Asian ginseng has an incredibly long history of use in medicine, dating back some six thousand years, and is valued especially for its restorative and energizing properties.

American ginseng has properties similar to those of Asian ginseng, but it is considered milder and is more likely to be prescribed for younger people.

Ginseng of either variety helps the body better utilize oxygen, spares glycogen utilization, increases cerebral circulation, helps the adrenal glands to better conserve their stores of vitamin C, aids in stabilizing blood sugar levels, helps balance hormone levels in men and women, and aids in the production of DNA and RNA. It helps the body adapt to stress and maintain normal blood pressure, glucose levels, and hormonal function.

It can improve energy, alertness, stamina, reaction time, and concentration, which makes it useful for such pursuits as studying, taking tests, long-distance driving, and meditating. It also speeds recovery time from sickness, surgery, childbirth, athletic performance, and other stressors to the body.

Although the root is the primary medicinal component of the plant, the leaves of both varieties can be used to treat hangover and fever.

Considerations

For best effect, take ginseng between meals rather than with food. It is best not to take ginseng at night, as it could impair sleep.

Avoid ginseng in cases of heat and inflammation, such as fever, flu, pneumonia, hypertension, or constipation. Do not give to children for prolonged periods, as it may cause early sexual maturation. Avoid during pregnancy and while nursing. Do not take ginseng in conjunction with cardiac glycosides except under the guidance of a qualified health care professional. Avoid for those with biploar conditions, as it may trigger mania.

GOTU KOLA

Botanical name: *Centella asiatica*
Family: Apiaceae (Parsley)
Part used: aboveground plant

Physiological Effects

Adaptogen, analgesic, antibacterial, anti-inflammatory, antioxidant, antirheumatic, antiseptic, antispasmodic, astringent, brain tonic, circulatory stimulant, decongestant, demulcent, depurative, endocrine tonic, hypotensive, immune tonic, laxative, nervine, rejuvenative, tonic, vasodilator, vulnerary

Medicinal Uses

In Asia gotu kola has long been considered a longevity tonic. An old Sinhalese proverb says of gotu kola, "Two leaves a day will keep old age away." And there are legends of a Chinese herbalist, Li Ching Yun, who supposedly consumed gotu kola regularly and lived to be 256 years old.

Gotu kola is known to regulate serotonin and dopamine levels in the brain, strengthen the body's membranes, help restore strength to the venous walls and connective tissue, improve neural transport, and help the body detoxify. It can be used to improve memory, calm anxiety, and alleviate depression. In traditional ayurvedic medicine it is used to balance the left and right sides of the brain.

Gotu kola is often taken as a brain tonic. On the first day of spring in Nepal, for example, gotu kola leaves are traditionally given to schoolchildren to improve their concentration and memory.

Considerations
Large doses can cause headache, itching, stupor, and vertigo. Avoid during pregnancy, except under the guidance of a qualified health care practitioner. Avoid in cases of overactive thyroid.

HAWTHORN

Botanical name: *Crataegus* spp.
Family: Rosaceae (Rose)
Parts used: leaf, flower, berry

Physiological Effects
Adaptogen, anabolic, anthelmintic, antibacterial, antioxidant, antispasmodic, cardiotonic, carminative, circulatory stimulant, digestive, diuretic, hypotensive, lithotriptic, nervine, nutritive, rejuvenative, sedative or stimulant (dose dependent), vasodilator, yin tonic

Medicinal Uses
Hawthorn strengthens the heart muscles, dilates the blood vessels, and improves circulation, including in the brain. Energetically, it calms the spirit.

Energetically, hawthorn promotes the healing power of hope, love, trust, and forgiveness. It helps relieve negative feelings from the heart and encourages knowledge of the strength and resiliency of the heart.

Considerations

Using hawthorn may potentiate the effects of heart medications such as beta-blockers or digoxin. If you are using heart medication, consult with a qualified health care professional before commencing use of hawthorn.

Use hawthorn with caution in cases of poor digestion or acid stomach. Hawthorn's effects are slow to manifest; the herb may need to be taken for four to eight weeks before results are observed. It is generally considered extremely safe.

HOPS

Botanical name: *Humulus lupulus*
Family: Cannabaceae (Hemp)
Part used: strobile (female inflorescence)

Physiological Effects

Anaphrodisiac, anodyne, antibiotic, anti-inflammatory, antiseptic, antispasmodic, aperient, astringent, cholagogue, diuretic, galactagogue, hypnotic, lithotriptic, muscle relaxant, nervine, sedative, soporific, stomachic

Medicinal Uses

Hops clears heat and toxins, nourishes yin, restrains infection, aids digestion, calms the spirit, stabilizes the nerves, eases anxiety, calms hyperactivity, and encourages sleep. Hops contains lupulin, which is considered a strong but safe, reliable sedative. If you don't react well to valerian, hops can be a good substitute.

Considerations

Avoid during pregnancy and in cases of depression. Use in conjunction with pharmaceutical sedatives only under the guidance of a qualified health care professional, as it may exacerbate their effects.

Fresh hops plants may cause contact dermatitis and allergic reactions in some individuals, and tiny hairs from the plant can irritate the eyes if they come in contact with them.

KAVA KAVA

Botanical name: *Piper methysticum*
Family: Piperaceae (Pepper)
Parts used: root, upper rhizome

Physiological Effects

Analgesic, anaphrodisiac (if used excessively), anesthetic, antifungal, antibacterial, anti-inflammatory, antiseptic, antispasmodic, aphrodisiac, diaphoretic, diuretic, euphoric, hypnotic, muscle relaxant, nervine, psychoactive, sedative, siliagogue, soporific, stimulant, tonic

Medicinal Uses

Kava kava is a traditional Polynesian remedy for insomnia and nervousness. It is often used in the islands ceremoniously, in religious rituals and rites to welcome guests and honor births, marriages, and business deals. It helps foster open communication and a feeling of letting go. It is also used for divination and to produce inspiration.

Kava kava helps warm the emotions, and small amounts can produce a pleasant, euphoric sensation. It calms nerves and respiration, reduces blood clotting, relaxes the muscles without blocking nerve signals, and eases physical tension without numbing mental processes. Taking kava kava before bed can help induce pleasant sleep and vivid dreams.

Kava kava is also said to increase tolerance of pain; Aborigines traditionally took kava kava before being tattooed, and women in labor sometimes drink kava kava juice as a calmative and to facilitate birth.

Kava kava can be used to ease anger, anxiety, mild depression, fear, nervousness, pain, and restlessness. It also takes the edge off withdrawal symptoms (from alcohol, nicotine, or tranquilizers).

Many constituents in kava kava are fat soluble, so when preparing it as a tea, add coconut milk to the steeping solution to help the infusion assimilate kava's compounds.

Considerations

Avoid during pregnancy and while nursing, and do not give to young children. Avoid in cases of Parkinson's disease and severe depression. Do not take in conjunction with alcohol, sedatives, tranquilizers, or antidepressants, as it can potentiate their effects.

Remain aware of kava kava's soporific effects; try to avoid driving, operating heavy machinery, or other activities that require fast reaction times after taking kava kava. On the plus side, kava kava, unlike many sedatives, is not habit forming. Daily use of kava shouldn't exceed three months, though occasional use on an ongoing basis is fine for those in good health.

Kava kava may cause the tongue, mouth, and other body parts to feel somewhat numb and rubbery temporarily; this is normal. However, excess amounts can cause disturbed vision, dilated pupils, and difficulty walking. Large doses taken for extended periods can have a cumulative effect on the liver, causing kavaism, a condition marked by a yellowish tinge to the skin, a scaly rash, apathy, anorexia, and bloodshot eyes.

There have been some reports of severe liver damage resulting from use of kava kava, prompting a number of nations to ban sales of it. The problem turned out to be caused by a compound called pipermethystine, found in the stem peelings and leaves of the kava plant but not in the roots. Traditional kava preparations are extracted from the roots, and the peelings and leaves are discarded. For this reason, avoid kava products made from the leaves or stems of the plant. The traditional tea prepared from the root appears to be quite safe.

LAVENDER

Botanical name: *Lavandula* spp., including *L. angustifolia,*
L. stoechas (French lavender), and *L. viridis*
Family: Lamiaceae (Mint)
Part used: flower

Physiological Effects

Analgesic, anaphrodisiac, antibacterial, antidepressant, antifungal, anti-inflammatory, antiseptic, antispasmodic, aromatic, bitter, carminative, cholagogue, digestive, diuretic (mild), expectorant, nervine, rubefacient, sedative, stimulant, tonic

Medicinal Uses

Lavender clears heat, calms nerves, and settles digestion. It is perhaps most popular for its spirit-lifting, nerve-relaxing, calming fragrance. Simply inhaling the scent of lavender essential oil from the bottle helps prevent fainting and relieves stress and depression. Lavender can be used to treat anxiety, mild depression, fear, headache (tension or migraine), insomnia, irritability, nervousness, pain, restlessness, and stress.

Considerations

Avoid large doses of lavender during pregnancy, as its effect on the developing fetus has not yet been determined.

LEMON BALM

Botanical name: *Melissa officinalis*
Family: Lamiaceae (Mint)
Part used: aboveground plant

Physiological Effects

Antidepressant, antihistamine, anti-inflammatory, antioxidant, antispasmodic, antiviral, aromatic, carminative, cephalic, cholagogue, hypotensive (mild), nervine, rejuvenative, sedative, stomachic, tonic, vasodilator

Medicinal Uses

Lemon balm, also called melissa, was widely used in ancient Greece and Rome. Avicenna, the great Arabic physician (980–1037), said that lemon balm caused "the mind and heart to be merry."

Lemon balm clears heat, calms the heart, improves concentration, cleanses the liver, improves chi circulation, lifts the spirits, and protects the brain from excessive stimuli. It eases anxiety and nervousness and helps with insomnia and fatigue. It is an uplifting bath herb. The essential oil can be inhaled several times daily to ease mild depression and help balance emotions.

It is a good herb for children; a cup of tea before bed can help prevent nightmares and allow for a good night's sleep, and it is excellent to calm the nerves and boost the mood of schoolchildren who are anxious about upcoming tests.

Considerations

Lemon balm is generally considered very safe and is a favorite herb for children. It can lower thyroid function, however, which is beneficial in some cases but not for those with a hypothyroid condition.

LICORICE

Botanical name: *Glycyrrhiza glabra* (European licorice), *G. lepidota* (American licorice), *G. inflata, G. uralensis* (Chinese licorice)
Family: Apiaceae (Parsley)
Part used: root (stolon)

Physiological Effects

Adrenal tonic, alterative, antacid, antiarthritic, antibacterial, antifungal, anti-inflammatory, antimutagenic, antioxidant, antiseptic, antispasmodic, antiviral, aperient, aphrodisiac, chi tonic, demulcent, emollient, expectorant, nutritive, phytoestrogenic, rejuvenative, sedative, sialogogue, tonic

Medicinal Uses

Licorice is one of the most commonly used herbs in traditional Chinese medicine. It harmonizes the effects of other herbs, helping to prolong their actions. It induces a feeling of calmness, peace, and harmony; it also slows the response to stress and relieves exhaustion caused by stress.

Considerations

Avoid licorice in cases of edema, nausea, vomiting, and rapid heartbeat. Licorice is not recommended during pregnancy or in combination with steroid or digoxin medications. Large doses may cause sodium retention and potassium depletion and may be emetic. Prolonged or excessive use may elevate blood pressure and cause headache and vertigo. Continuous use is not recommended in excess of six weeks, except under the guidance of a qualified health care practitioner.

Chinese licorice (*G. uralensis*) is said to be less likely to cause side effects than the European variety (*G. glabra*). All these precautions notwithstanding, licorice is often added in very small amounts to other herbal medicines, so if you are at risk, read the label.

LINDEN

Botanical name: *Tilia* spp., including *T. americana,*
T. cordata, T. x *europea,* and *T. platyphyllos*
Family: Tiliaceae (Tilia)
Part used: flower

Physiological Effects

Antidepressant, antispasmodic, cephalic, cholagogue, choleretic, diaphoretic, diuretic, emollient, expectorant, hypotensive, nervine, sedative, stomachic, sudorific, tonic, vasodilator, vulnerary

Medicinal Uses

Linden moves stagnant chi, calms the nerves, and promotes rest. It also helps heal blood vessel walls, and its high mucilage content helps soothe irritated respiratory passages. It is used in the treatment of anxiety, headache, hypertension, hysteria, indigestion, insomnia, migraine, pain, and stress. As a bath herb, it promotes relaxation and is often used to calm restless children.

Considerations

Tilia americana should be consumed in moderation, as large doses may cause nausea.

LION'S MANE MUSHROOM

Botanical name: *Hericium erinaceus*
Family: Hericiaceae
Parts used: fruiting body, mycelium

Physiological Effects

Anti-inflammatory, antioxidant, hypolipidemic, immune tonic, neuroptotective, neuroregenerative

Medicinal Uses

Lion's mane appears to decrease the amyloid plaque buildup in the brain that can contribute to cognitive decline. It stimulates neural growth and rebuilding of the myelin nerve sheath, and it has been found to increase the production of nerve growth factor (NGF), which is imperative for the forebrain's cholinergic system. It also promotes strength and vigor. It is being used to treat Alzheimer's, anxiety, brain injury, cognitive impairment, depression, inflammation, and Parkinson's.

Considerations

There are no known side effects beyond the occasional itchy skin due to nerve growth. The mushrooms have a long history of culinary and medicinal use in Asia; they can be consumed as a food (cooked, rather than raw) as well as a supplement.

MILK THISTLE

Botanical name: *Silybum marianum*
Family: Asteraceae (Daisy)
Part used: seed

Physiological Effects

Antidepressant, antioxidant, appetite stimulant, astringent, bitter tonic, cholagogue, demulcent, hepatoprotective, stomachic, tonic

Medicinal Uses

Milk thistle seed helps protect the liver, prevents toxins from penetrating liver cells, promotes the growth of healthy liver cells, and improves the liver's function. It offers excellent support for the liver for those who need to take pharmaceutical drugs.

Considerations

There have been occasional reports of the seeds causing bloating or diarrhea or having a laxative effect.

MOTHERWORT

Botanical name: *Leonurus cardiaca*
Family: Lamiaceae (Mint)
Part used: aboveground plant (including the seed)

Physiological Effects

Analgesic, antibacterial, antifungal, antioxidant, antirheumatic, antispasmodic, astringent, cardiotonic, circulatory stimulant, emmenagogue, hemostatic, hypotensive, immune stimulant, laxative, nervine, sedative, stomachic, tonic, vasodilator

Medicinal Uses

Motherwort slows a rapid heartbeat, improves circulation, prevents blood platelet aggregation, regulates the menstrual cycle, and calms anxiety and stress that may contribute to heart problems. It is especially beneficial to women's health. It's said to make mothers more joyful and modulates tendencies to "overmother."

Considerations

Avoid motherwort in cases of excessive menstrual bleeding. Avoid during pregnancy (but note that motherwort can be helpful during labor, under the guidance of a qualified health care professional).

NETWORK
NETTLE

Botanical name: *Urtica dioica, U. urens*
Family: Urticaceae (Nettle)
Part used: aboveground plant

Physiological Effects

Adrenal tonic, alterative, antiallergenic, antihistamine, anti-inflammatory, antioxidant, antirheumatic, blood tonic, cholagogue, circulatory stimulant, hypoglycemic, kidney tonic, lithotriptic, nervine, nutritive

Medicinal Uses

This herb improves just about everything! As David Hoffmann, author of *The Holistic Herbal,* says, "When in doubt, use nettles."

Nettle improves the body's resistance to pollens, molds, and environmental pollutants. It stabilizes mast cell walls, which stops the cycle of mucous membrane hyperactivity, and it nourishes and tones the veins, improves veins' elasticity, and reduces inflammation. It is a COX-2 inhibitor. Nettle is considered a nervine or restorative for the nervous system and the brain. It is rich in silica which is also a component of the nerve sheaths in the body, making nettles a beneficial remedy for stress, nervousness, and depression.

It also helps cleanses toxins from the body, energizes, and curbs appetite. Drinking nettle tea before and after surgery helps build the blood, promotes healthy blood clotting (due to its vitamin K content), speeds recovery, and helps the patient reclaim their energy. Nettle is a highly nutritious, blood-building herb that is particularly strengthening to the kidneys. Nettle is also a traditional folk remedy for feelings of panic and powerlessness and has long been suggested for those exhibiting poor concentration, poor memory, dullness, and difficulty getting up or being motivated.

Considerations

All fifty species of the genus *Urtica* can be used medicinally, but stick with the *urens* and *dioica* species unless you have consulted with local herb authorities on the safety of local varieties.

Nettle is not known as stinging nettle for nothing; avoid touching or eating the fresh plant unless it is very young and/or you are very brave. Touching the fresh plant can cause a burning rash. Wearing gloves when collecting can help prevent this, but the hairs in large plants may still pierce through. A nettle sting can be soothed with a poultice of yellow dock or plantain. However, in ancient times nettle sting was used therapeutically to increase circulation to specific areas, including paralyzed limbs.

Eating raw nettles can cause digestive disturbances, mouth and lip irritation, and urinary problems; however, these side effects are rare when the plant is pureed before ingestion and practically nonexistent when the plant is dried. When used appropriately, nettle is considered safe, even over an extended period of time, although those with overly cold, yin-deficient conditions should not use nettle for prolonged periods.

OAT

Botanical name: *Avena fatua* (wild oat),
A. sativa (cultivated oat)
Family: Poaceae (Grass)
Parts used: seed (unripe), stem (oatstraw)

Physiological Effects

Alterative, antidepressant, antispasmodic, aphrodisiac, blood tonic, brain tonic, chi tonic, demulcent, diaphoretic, diuretic, emollient, endocrine tonic, febrifuge, laxative, mood elevator, nervine, nervous system tonic, nutritive, rejuvenative, reproductive tonic, restorative

Medicinal Uses

The alkaloids in oat nourish the limbic system and motor ganglia, increasing energy levels and a sense of well-being. With its high silicon content, oat helps nourish the skin, nails, teeth, bones, and hair. It builds the blood, relaxes the nerves, and strengthens the nervous system, making tactile sensations more pleasurable. It supports treatment of addiction, alcoholism, anxiety, mild depression, exhaustion, insomnia, nervousness, and post-traumatic stress. When consumed regularly, oat can lower cholesterol levels.

As a flower essence, Wild Oat is helpful for those who are filled with uncertainty and dissatisfaction and are unable to find their life's direction.

Considerations

Those with gluten allergies should use oat with caution.

PASSIONFLOWER

Botanical name: *Passiflora* spp., including
P. edulis (yellow passionflower) and *P. incarnata*
Family: Passifloraceae (Passionflower)
Parts used: leaf, vine, flower

Physiological Effects

Analgesic, anodyne, antibacterial, antidepressant, antifungal, anti-inflammatory, antispasmodic, antitussive, aphrodisiac, cerebral vasorelaxant, diaphoretic, diuretic, hypnotic, hypotensive, nervine, sedative

Medicinal Uses

Passionflower calms the central nervous system, slows the breakdown of serotonin and norepinephrine, induces a mild euphoria, and quiets mental chatter and anxiety. It also promotes peaceful sleep. Choose passionflower to relieve anger, anxiety, irritability, stress, worry, and restlessness. It's safe even for children and the elderly.

Passionflower helps us integrate spirituality into daily life. It also helps clear emotional confusion and relieves pain and the after-effects of trauma.

Considerations

Large doses may cause nausea and vomiting. Avoid large doses during pregnancy. Unripe fruits have some level of toxicity and should not be consumed.

PSILOCYBIN MUSHROOMS

Botanical name: There are more than a hundred different
species of mushrooms that contain psilocybin.
Some of the better-known ones are:

Conocybe cyanopus	*Psilocybe bohemica*
Inocybe aeruginascens	*Psilocybe cubensis*

Panaeolus africanus	*Psilocybe cyanescens*
Panaeolus cinctulus	*Psilocybe mexicana*
Panaeolus cyanescens	*Psilocybe semilanceata*
Psilocybe azurescens	*Psilocybe tampanensis*

Family: Polyporaceae (Polypor)
Part used: fruiting body

Physiological Effects

Analgesic, anti-inflammatory, antioxidant, neuroregenerative, psychoactive

Medicinal Effects

Psilocybin mushrooms are a group of mushrooms that contain psilocybin. Upon ingestion, the body converts psilocybin to psilocin, a psychoactive compound. Indigenous peoples across North and South America used these mushrooms in religious and healing ceremonies. The Aztec referred them as *teonanacatl,* or flesh of the gods.

Psilocybin activates specific dopamine pathways in the brain and boosts levels of serotonin, and the resulting effects include altered perceptions, euphoria, hallucinations, relaxation, and visual enhancements of color and light.

By altering consciousness, psilocybin allows access to the subconscious and can help resolve issues of addiction, anxiety, depression, obsessive-compulsive disorder, and post-traumatic stress. Psilocybin-assisted psychotherapy has been shown to reduce anxiety and improve mood without clinically significant adverse effects.

Considerations

Nausea, vomiting, euphoria, muscle weakness or relaxation, drowsiness, and lack of coordination may occur. Psilocybin mushrooms are not appropriate for use by people with psychotic disorders. They should not be used by anyone who is taking SSRI or MAOI drugs, and they should not be combined with alcohol. Avoid during pregnancy, and use only with great caution in cases of diabetes.

REISHI

Botanical name: *Ganoderma lucidum*
Family: Polyporaceae (Polypor)
Part used: fruiting body

Physiological Effects

Adaptogen, analgesic, antibacterial, anti-inflammatory, antioxidant, antitumor, antitussive, antiviral, cardiotonic, expectorant, hepatoprotective, hypotensive, immune stimulant, rejuvenative

Medicinal Uses

Reishi is considered a longevity herb in Chinese medicine and has been in use in that tradition for more than four thousand years. In the Taoist tradition, reishi is said to enhance spiritual receptivity, and it is used by monks to calm the spirit and mind. It is known to normalize blood pressure and blood sugar levels, lower levels of low-density lipoproteins (LDL, or "bad" cholesterol), and inhibit histamine release and blood platelet aggregation. It also activates the phagocytosis of macrophages and stimulates interferon production and activity, thereby supporting the immune system, and inhibits the activity of staphyloccus and streptococcus.

Reishi is used in the treatment of allergies, arthritis, cancer, depression, diabetes, fatigue, food sensitivities, high cholesterol, hypertension, hypotension, insomnia, nephritis, and stroke.

Considerations

Reishi has a very low potential for toxicity. When pregnant or while nursing, use only under the guidance of a qualified health care practitioner. Long-term use may cause dry mouth, dizziness, and digestive distress. Because reishi can inhibit blood clotting, it should be avoided for at least one week before surgery, before childbirth, or in conjunction with blood-thinning medications.

RHODIOLA

Botanical name: *Rhodiola rosea*
Family: Crassulaceae (Stonecrop)
Part used: root

Physiological Effects

Adaptogen, anti-inflammatory, antioxidant, nootropic, stimulant, stomachic, tonic

Medicinal Uses

Rhodiola inhibits the breakdown of neurotransmitters, including serotonin and dopamine; it has been found to increase serotonin levels in the brain by up to 30 percent. It also increases mental and physical performance; it can shorten recovery time between athletic endeavors, such as workouts, and can improve memory and work productivity. In Siberia it is traditionally given to couples prior to marriage to help them bring forth healthy children.

Rhodiola is used in the treatment of anxiety, depression, erectile dysfunction, exhaustion, fatigue, headache, hysteria, insomnia, stress, nervous system disorders, pain, premature ejaculation, and stress.

Considerations

Rhodiola is generally regarded as safe.

ROSEMARY

Botanical name: *Rosmarinus officinalis*
Family: Lamiaceae (Mint)
Part used: aboveground plant

Physiological Effects

Anodyne, antibacterial, antidepressant, antifungal, anti-inflammatory, antioxidant, antiseptic, antispasmodic, aromatic, cephalic, cholagogue, choleretic, circulatory stimulant, diaphoretic, hypertensive, nervine, ophthalmic, rejuvenative, rubefacient, stimulant, stomachic, yang tonic

Medicinal Uses

Rosemary has a delightful aroma and a long European tradition of use in alleviating anxiety. It inhibits COX-2-related inflammation, stimulates the pineal gland, improves energy levels, and relieves stress. Rosemary contains the nutrients calcium, magnesium, potassium, phosphorus, iron, and potassium as well as more than a dozen antioxidants. It can be used to treat dull, lethargic depression, where life seems too much of a bother and you feel like you're in a mental fog.

In the bath, rosemary rejuvenates the body and mind and helps relieve pain and sore muscles.

Considerations

Avoid therapeutic doses during pregnancy (though using rosemary moderately to season food is safe). Though rosemary is generally considered so safe that it is a common kitchen herb, extremely large doses could cause convulsions and death.

SAINT JOHN'S WORT

Botanical name: *Hypericum* spp., including *H. perforatum*
Family: Clusiaceae (Saint John's Wort)
Part used: flowering top

Physiological Effects

Alterative, analgesic, anodyne, antidepressant, anti-inflammatory, antioxidant, antiseptic, antispasmodic, anxiolytic, astringent, cholagogue, digestive, diuretic, expectorant, nerve restorative, sedative, vermifuge, vulnerary

Medicinal Uses

Saint John's wort has been used for more than a thousand years to treat depression. Its action results in part from its ability to block the reabsorption of serotonin, and it may also enhance the body's receptivity to light. One of its constituents, hypericin, increases serotonin and melatonin metabolism. Another component, hyperforin, inhibits the uptake of dopamine, serotonin, noradrenaline, gamma-aminobutyric acid (GABA), and L-glutamate, thereby allowing these neurotransmitters to persist longer in the body, which contributes to emotional stability.

It can help heal damaged nerves when used internally or externally. It also promotes tissue repair, deters infection, and helps relieve pain.

This herb benefits anxiety, mild to moderate depression, fear, irritability, chronic fatigue, obsessive-compulsive disorder, migraine, and fibromyalgia. It has been known to restore zest to the elderly who feel lonely and uncared for.

Topically, Saint John's wort can be prepared as a compress to treat pain, and nerve pain. The oil or liniment can be used for massaging the spine, neck, and head in cases of neurological damage, arthritis, neuralgia, and sciatica.

Saint John's wort's effects are not instantaneous. Continued use is necessary, and as many as two to six weeks may be needed before the herb's effects manifest.

Considerations

Saint John's wort should not be combined with antidepressant pharmaceuticals, protease inhibitors, MAOIs, or organ antirejection drugs (such as cyclosporine), except under the guidance of a qualified health care practitioner. In fact, because Saint John's wort cleanses the liver, where many old stored emotions are said to reside, it is best to use it with caution in conjunction with any pharmaceutical drug.

Saint John's wort is not recommended for anyone who is pregnant or breastfeeding or for children under the age of two. It may cause photosensitivity, especially in fair-skinned individuals. There have been rare reports of dizziness, nausea, fatigue, and dry mouth from its use. Some people may experience contact dermatitis from the plant.

SCHISANDRA

Botanical name: *Schisandra chinensis, S. sphenanthera*
Family: Schisandraceae (Magnolia Vine)
Part used: berry

Physiological Effects

Adaptogen, antidepressant, antioxidant, aphrodisiac, astringent, brain tonic, cholagogue, hepatoprotective, immune tonic, kidney tonic, nervous system tonic, rejuvenative, reproductive tonic, restorative, sedative (mild), yang tonic, yin tonic

Medicinal Uses

Schisandra was widely used by the royalty of ancient China as a youth preserver, beautifier, and reproductive tonic. It is a supreme adaptogen; Russian pilots of the 1940s used it to help them tolerate the low-oxygen conditions of high altitudes, while to this day hunters in Siberia consume schisandra berries for energy and to help their bodies function in the harsh conditions.

Schisandra quickens reflex time, stabilizes the nervous system, normalizes brain function, and improves coordination, intellect, and sensory perception. Chinese medicine calls for eating a few berries one hundred days in a row as a tonic to improve coordination and concentration. According to Chinese theory, schisandra also helps build your defensive energy, or *wei chi,* so you are better able to resist infection. Schisandra is both astringent and demulcent, having the ability to both dry and moisten as needed. It is used to nourish the "water of the genitals," or the fluids that help sensitize and moisturize the genitals. Long-term use helps beautify the skin.

Schisandra berries are used in the treatment of anxiety, cerebral ataxia, cirrhosis, chronic fatigue syndrome, depression, diabetes, dizziness, exhaustion, headache, heart palpitations, insomnia, irritability, memory loss, nephritis, neuralgia, neuroses, Parkinson's disease, posttraumatic stress disorder, stress, and wasting diseases. It also can facilitate athletic recovery and improve sexual stamina.

Considerations

Avoid schisandra in cases of excess heat (such as fever), overly acidic conditions, cough, epilepsy, intracranial pressure, or the early stages of rash. Schisandra is not recommended during pregnancy. Do not give to children under the age of two, except under the guidance of a qualified health care practitioner.

SKULLCAP

Botanical name: *Scutellaria californica, S. elliptica, S. galericulata, S. incana, S. lateriflora, S. ovata, S. tuberosa*
Family: Lamiaceae (Mint)
Part used: aboveground plant

Physiological Effects

Anaphrodisiac, anodyne, antibacterial, antispasmodic, brain tonic, cardiotonic, cerebral vasodilator, hypotensive, nervine, nervous system tonic, restorative, sedative, spinal cord tonic, stomachic

Medicinal Uses

Skullcap calms and strengthens the nerves, relaxes spasms, relieves pain, and promotes rest. It can help rebuild myelin nerve sheaths. One of its constituents, scutellarin, is transformed in the body into scutellarein, which helps stimulate the brain to produce more endorphins.

Skullcap is used to treat addiction, anger, anxiety, attention deficit disorder, chorea, convulsions, delirium, emotional upset, epilepsy, fear, headache, high cholesterol, hypertension, hysteria, insomnia, multiple sclerosis, muscle cramps, nervous exhaustion, nervous stomach, neuralgia, pain, palsy, panic attacks, Parkinson's disease, premenstrual syndrome, restlessness, rheumatism, spasms, tremors, and withdrawal symptoms (from alcohol, drugs, and tobacco).

Skullcap works best when given over a period of time. It loses its properties more quickly than many herbs; herb stock that is more than a year old is not likely to have much therapeutic value.

Skullcap promotes relaxation and can be helpful for those who are preoccupied. It also aids in withdrawal from drugs, especially opiates.

Contraindications
Avoid during pregnancy. Large doses may cause confusion and giddiness.

TEA, GREEN

Botanical name: *Camellia sinensis*
Family: Theaceae (Tea)
Parts used: leaf bud, young leaf

Physiological Effects
Analgesic, antibacterial, antioxidant, antiseptic, antiviral, astringent, cardiotonic, hypotensive, immune stimulant, nervine, stimulant

Medicinal Uses
Of the three most common types of tea—black, green, and oolong—green tea contains the most polyphenols, at about 15 to 30 percent by weight. About half of that is epigallocatechin gallate (EGCG). Tea's polyphenols, and especially EGCG, are recognized as antioxidants. EGCG has been found to be twenty times stronger than vitamin E in protecting brain lipids, which are very susceptible to oxidative stress.

Green tea also prevents blood platelet aggregation, the "clumping together" of blood that can lead to blood clots, heart attacks, and stroke. Its polyphenols, along with its vitamin C content, also help strengthen blood vessel walls. In fact, the consumption of green tea with meals has been shown to reduce the occurrence of arterial disease, and a study of six thousand Japanese women found that those who drank about five cups of green tea daily had a 50 percent decrease in the risk of stroke.

Whereas coffee can elevate cholesterol levels, green tea helps lower them. The catechin content of green tea helps break down cholesterol and increase its elimination through the bowels. Green tea also helps keep blood sugar levels moderate.

Green tea has about 25 mg of caffeine per cup (about one-third to half as much as a cup of coffee). Caffeine blocks the naturally occurring tranquilizer adenosine, so that the brain becomes stimulated. It also increases the synthesis of catecholamines, which relay nerve impulses in the brain. It is believed that the constituent tannins and vitamin C help moderate the effects of caffeine in tea, so that the deleterious side effects—jitteriness, irritability, and (after the effect has worn off) fatigue—are minimal compared to other caffeine sources, which may explain why Zen monks rely on green tea to help them remain alert yet calm during long periods of meditation.

Many of tea's other constituents have been and are being studied. One of the widely researched components in tea is the alkaloid theanine; it is an amino acid that has been found to decrease anxiety, aid in sleep, and promote mental focus.

Considerations

Excessive use of tea may cause nervous irritability and digestive distress such as ulcers. Avoid tea in cases of hypertension and insomnia; avoid large doses during pregnancy and while nursing.

TURMERIC

Botanical name: *Curcuma longa*
Family: Zingiberaceae (Ginger)
Part used: rhizome

Physiological Effects

Analgesic, antifungal, anti-inflammatory, antioxidant, antiseptic, cholagogue, choleretic, circulatory stimulant, emmenagogue, hepatoprotective, hepatotonic, hypoglycemic, stimulant, stomachic, vulnerary

Medicinal Uses

Turmeric is one of the best and safest anti-inflammatory agents, largely due to its constituent alkaloid curcumin. It sensitizes the body's cortisol receptor sites, inhibits COX-2 and 5-LOX enzymes, and reduces platelet aggregation. It even reduces amyloid plaque buildups in the brain. It also helps stabilize the body's microflora, thus inhibiting yeast overgrowth. It is used in the treatment of arthritis, asthma, cancer, candida, depression, eczema, gastritis, high cholesterol, jaundice, memory loss, nausea, and trauma.

Considerations

Avoid therapeutic dosages during pregnancy (though culinary use is fine). Turmeric may cause photosensitivity in some individuals. It may also cause contact dermatitis in rare cases. The addition of piperine, a compound found in black pepper, may increase turmeric's bioavailability.

VALERIAN

Botanical name: *Valeriana* spp., including *V. officinalis*
Family: Valerianaceae (Valerian)
Parts used: root, rhizome

Physiological Effects

Anodyne, antibacterial, antispasmodic, hypnotic, hypotensive, nervous system tonic, nervine, restorative, sedative, smooth muscle relaxant, stomachic, tonic

Medicinal Effect

Valerian is sometimes referred to as a "daytime sedative" because it can improve performance, concentration, and memory during the day and help you sleep better during the night, including reducing the time needed to fall asleep. It calms nerves and eases anxiety and panic without dulling the mind. Its effects are due to one of its constituents, valerenic acid, which has been shown to inhibit the action of the enzyme that breaks down GABA (gamma-aminobutyric acid), thus contributing to increased levels of calming GABA in the body.

Valerian is used in the treatment of addiction (tobacco or tranquilizer), aggressiveness (chronic), anxiety, arthritis pain, ADHD, chorea, convulsions, delirium tremens, dysmenorrhea, epilepsy, headache, hypertension (due to stress), hyperactivity, hypochondria, hysteria, inflammatory bowel disorder, insomnia, mental illness, migraine, muscle pain, nervousness, nervous breakdown, neuralgia, pain, premenstrual syndrome, restlessness during illness, shock, stress, and traumatic injury.

Topically, valerian can be used as a poultice to relieve pain.

Considerations

Large doses of valerian can cause depression, nausea, headache, and lethargy. Some individuals, especially those who are already overheated, may find valerian stimulating rather than sedating. Do not use large doses for more than three weeks in a row. Avoid during pregnancy, except in very small doses. Do not give to children under the age of three. Avoid in cases of very low blood pressure or hypoglycemia; avoid long-term use in cases of depression.

Use with caution if you are going to be driving, operating heavy machinery, or undertaking other activities that require fast reaction times.

Valerian may potentiate the effects of benzodiazepine and barbiturates. Those taking sedatives, antidepressants, or antianxiety medications should use valerian only under the guidance of a qualified health care professional.

Note: Avoid boiling the root when making tea, which would diminish the plant's activity.

Many find the aroma of valerian unpleasant, much like that of dirty socks. Some find that making valerian tea with raisins added to the water improves the flavor. Or you can rely on capsules or tinctures instead of tea.

WILD LETTUCE

Botanical name: *Lactuca canadensis,*
L. serriola (prickly lettuce), *L. virosa* (bitter lettuce)
Family: Asteraceae (Daisy)
Parts used: leaf, latex

Physiological Effects

Analgesic, anaphrodisiac, anodyne, antispasmodic, antitussive, digestive, diuretic, expectorant, febrifuge, galactagogue, hypnotic, hypoglycemic, narcotic, sedative

Medicinal Uses

Wild lettuce calms the nervous system, aids sleep, and relieves pain, anxiety, and restlessness. The dried leaves can be smoked or made into a tea to ease pain and calm stress. Wild lettuce contains a milky white latex that has euphoric properties, similar to opium, but without the addictive potential.

Considerations

Wild lettuce is best used only under the guidance of a qualified health care professional. Moderate doses can cause drowsiness, while large doses can give rise to excessive sexual urges or insomnia. Very large doses can be fatal.

The latex from the plant can cause eye irritation or contact dermatitis in some individuals.

WOOD BETONY

Botanical name: *Stachys hyssopifolia, S. officinalis,*
S. palustris (marsh betony), *S. sylvatica*
Family: Lamiaceae (Mint)
Part used: aboveground plant

Physiological Effects
Alterative, analgesic, antispasmodic, astringent, aromatic, bitter, carminative, cerebral tonic, circulatory stimulant, diuretic, hepatotonic, hypoglycemic, hypotensive, nervine, sedative (mild), styptic, vulnerary

Medicinal Uses
Wood betony strengthens the nerves and has a calming effect on them. It can help with anxiety, fear, stress, worry, and persistent unwanted thoughts and promotes a more positive outlook. It can help relieve pain, including headaches, migraines, and neuralgia.

Wood betony promotes deep rest, helping relieve insomnia, exhaustion, and nightmares. It breaks up chi stagnation and helps move stagnation in the liver and circulatory system.

Considerations
Wood betony is generally regarded as safe. However, large doses may cause vomiting. Pregnant women should avoid large doses, except during labor, and then only under the guidance of a qualified health care practitioner.

Do not confuse *Stachys* with another genus, *Pedicularis*, also known as betony, as their uses are not interchangeable.

YERBA MATÉ

Botanical name: *Ilex paraguariensis*
Family: Aquifoliaceae (Holly)
Part used: leaf

Physiological Effects

Alterative, antibacterial, antioxidant, antiscorbutic, antispasmodic, aperient, aphrodisiac, astringent, cardiotonic, depurative, diaphoretic, digestive, diuretic, immune stimulant, nervous system stimulant, purgative (in large amounts), rejuvenative, stimulant, stomachic, sudorific, thermogenic, tonic

Medicinal Uses

Yerba maté cleanses the blood, decreases the appetite, and stimulates the mind, the respiratory system, and the nervous system. It is said to help users better tolerate hot, humid weather. Because maté helps cleanse the body of wastes without harming beneficial intestinal flora, some people drink it when they are on a cleanse, diet, or fast. It is often used to improve memory and concentration. It also delays the buildup of uric acid after a workout, thereby improving motor response.

Yerba maté is used in the treatment of allergies, arthritis, constipation, depression, diabetes, fatigue, hay fever, headache, heavy metal toxicity, hypotension, migraines, neuralgia, obesity, rheumatic pain, sinusitis, and stress.

The tea's saponin and tannin content make it useful as a wash in cleansing wounds and as a compress to speed the healing process.

Considerations

Maté contains caffeine; however, its tannins tend to bind with the caffeine, thereby reducing both compounds' effects. Most people who find that caffeine impairs their sleep will not experience this effect with maté. But those suffering from anxiety, heart palpitations, or insomnia should use maté cautiously.

It is best to avoid consuming maté with meals, as the high tannin content can impair nutrient assimilation. Avoid drinking maté (or any beverage) extremely hot, as it can damage the esophagus.

Choosing Tea Herbs for Specific Uses

With just a small repertoire of herbs, you can create effective, safe, and delicious healing tea blends that nourish, cleanse, and support the body in a multitude of manners. (Note that all of the herbs listed here work well as teas but could also be taken in capsule or tincture form.)

Addiction-Free Teas

The following herbs help reduce cravings for harmful substances.

Basil	Fennel seed
Catnip	Lemon balm
Cinnamon	Oatstraw or oats
Clove	Orange peel
Dandelion root	Spearmint

Blood-Sugar-Stabilizing Teas

Help stabilize the highs and lows of blood glucose levels with these herbs.

Blueberries	Fennel seed
Burdock root	Fenugreek seed
Cinnamon	Marshmallow root
Dandelion root	

Brain Booster Teas

Sharpen your wits with classic smart herbs.

Ginkgo	Rosemary
Gotu kola	Sage
Nettle leaf	Yerba maté
Oatstraw or oats	

Calm Stress Teas

Sip a cup of soothing, stress-relieving tea.

Catnip	Lemon balm
Chamomile	Oatstraw or oats

Depression Uplift Teas

These herbs help raise your spirits when you feel blue.

Dandelion root	Oatstraw or oats
Goji berry	Saint John's wort
Lemon balm	Spearmint
Nettle	

Energy Teas

These herbs help you buzz around.

Green tea	Nettle
Hawthorn leaf and flower	Oatstraw or oats
Licorice root	Yerba maté

Get Grounded Teas

Get grounded with deep roots!

Burdock root	Ginger
Dandelion root	

Headache-Free Teas

These herbs help relieve the pain and inflammation
of a throbbing head.

Chamomile   Peppermint
Dandelion root   Rosemary
Lemon balm

Pain Relief Teas

The following herbs are analgesic, anti-inflammatory, and calming.

Chamomile   Marshmallow root
Clove   Peppermint
Linden flower   Rosemary

Recovery Teas

For recovery from surgery, accidents, illness, trauma, or grief,
turn to these nutritious, healing teas.

Dandelion root   Plantain leaf
Marshmallow root   Rose hips
Nettle   Violet leaf
Oatstraw or oats

Bedtime Teas

Soothe yourself to sleep with a nerve nourishing calming tea.

Catnip   Linden flower
Chamomile   Oatstraw or oats
Lemon balm

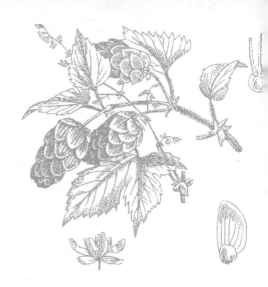

23
Essential
Nutrients

These are the nutrients that can best help support mental and emotional health and healing. The profiles here open with a brief discussion of each nutrient's actions and benefits, which is followed by a list of the foods in which each nutrient can be found. If you're looking to focus on a particular nutritional compound, be sure to eat adequate amounts of the foods listed with it. Of course, you must be sure to eat a wide range of foods in order to meet your body's overall nutritional requirements. Having a varied diet enables you to build an optimal nutritional foundation. Supplements can help boost your level of specific nutrients for improved health and wellness.

VITAMINS

Carotenoids (Vitamin A)

Carotenoids prevent vision problems, improve skin health, help repair the lining of the respiratory and digestive tracts, enhance immunity, and give protection against pollution. There are many different kinds. Monoterpene carotenoids, in addition to having these characteristics, are antioxidant and protect against cancer and heart disease.

Alpha-Carotene

Sources: apricot, berries, broccoli, carrots, corn, green leafy vegetables, oranges, peaches, pumpkins, seaweed, sweet potatoes

Beta-Carotene

Sources: apricots, bell peppers. broccoli, cabbage, cantaloupe, grapefruit, green leafy vegetables, lamb's-quarter, mangoes, nori, oranges, papayas, parsley, persimmons, pumpkins, sweet potatoes, tomatoes, watermelon, winter squash, yams, yellow.squash

Lutein

Benefits vision.

Sources: Beets, broccoli, Brussels sprouts, calendula flowers, carrots, collard greens, corn, dandelion blossoms, grapes (red), green leafy vegetables (kale, lettuce, spinach, turnip greens, etc.) hibiscus, kiwi, marigold flowers, mustard greens, orange juice, paprika, peas, potatoes, pumpkins, red peppers, spirulina, taro root, tomatoes, winter squash, zucchini

Lycopene

Source: Apricots, carrots, grapefruit (pink), grapes, green leafy vegetables, green peppers, guavas, kiwi, marigold flowers, oranges, papaya, paprika, spirulina, squash, tomatoes, watermelon, zucchini

Vitamin B Complex

These eight vitamins function as coenzymes and are especially important in the metabolism of fats, carbohydrates, and protein. B-complex vitamins are needed for cellular reproduction, including red and white blood cell production. Individual B vitamins also have unique benefits, which are described in the following pages. If you're taking a B-complex supplement, take it in the morning for increased energy and with food to prevent any digestive distress. All of the B vitamins, but especially B_6, have been linked to better brain function.

The B Complex

B_1 (thiamine)	B_6 (pyridoxine)
B_2 (riboflavin)	B_7 (biotin)
B_3 (niacin)	B_9 (folate/folic acid)
B_5 (pantothenic acid)	B_{12} (cobalamin)

Vitamin B_1 (Thiamine)

Thiamine is necessary for a sense of well-being. It promotes muscle tone in the digestive tract, improves nutrient assimilation, and stabilizes the appetite. A deficiency in B_1 can be a factor in poor memory, lack of coordination, dementia, irritability, and alcohol cravings. Use of alcohol and tobacco, as well as contraceptives, antacids, diuretics, sedatives, and some chemotherapy and antiseizure medications increase the body's need for thiamine.

Sources: apricots, asparagus, avocados, beans, beef, black beans, broccoli, brown rice, eggs, fish (tuna), green leafy vegetables, millet, nutritional yeast, nuts (all, but especially almonds, Brazil nuts, pine nuts, and pistachios), oatmeal, oranges, peas, pineapple, rye, seeds (chia, flax, hemp, pumpkin, sesame, sunflower), soy, watermelon, whole grains

Vitamin B_2 (Riboflavin)

Riboflavin supports growth and energy and promotes healthy vision, preventing dry eyes and cataracts. It is also needed for the health of skin, hair, and nails. Cracks around the corners of the mouth, fatigue, and weakness can indicate a riboflavin deficiency. Daily supplementation may help prevent migraines.

Sources: almonds, asparagus, avocados, beans, bee pollen and royal jelly, black currants, broccoli, dairy, eggs, green leafy vegetables (especially collard greens and spinach), meat, mushrooms, nutritional yeast, nuts, okra, rice, soy, sunflower seeds, whole grains

Vitamin B₃ (Niacin)

In addition to aiding the metabolism of fats, carbohydrates, and proteins, niacin helps regulate blood sugar levels, nourishes the nerves, and lowers cholesterol. This nutrient is necessary for the production of adrenal and sex hormones. It inhibits the breakdown of tryptophan, which, in turn, allows the synthesis of more serotonin. A niacin deficiency, known as pellagra, can contribute to depression, irritability, memory loss, disorientation, confusion, and insomnia.

Sources: anchovies, asparagus, avocado, barley, beans, bee pollen, broccoli, cantaloupe, carrots, chicken, dates, eggs, figs, fish (tuna), green leafy vegetables, liver, meat, millet, mushrooms, nutritional yeast, peanuts, prunes, raspberries, rice, salmon, sesame seeds, soybeans, squash, strawberries, sunflower seeds, tempeh, tomatoes, turkey, watermelon, whole grains

Vitamin B₅ (Pantothenic Acid)

Pantothenic acid is needed by the adrenal glands for hormone production and is important in energy production.

Sources: asparagus, avocado, beans (especially lentils and soybeans), bee pollen and royal jelly, broccoli, buckwheat, cabbage, corn, green leafy vegetables, meat, nutritional yeast, nuts (especially cashews, hazelnuts, and pecans), papayas, peas, pineapple, seeds (especially flax, hemp, sesame, and sunflower), salmon, shiitakes, watermelon, whole grains

Vitamin B₆ (Pyridoxine)

Pyridoxine is important for hormonal balance and is required for the production of stomach acids and the absorption of vitamin B₁₂. It also supports immune system function and helps make norepinephrine and serotonin.

Sources: apples, asparagus, avocado, bananas, barley, beans (especially garbanzo, lentils, lima, navy, soybeans), beef liver, bee pollen, blueberries, brown rice, buckwheat, cabbage, cantaloupe, carrots, chicken, corn, eggs, fish (tuna), flaxseed, green leafy vegetables, mangoes, mushrooms, nutritional yeast, nuts (Brazil nuts, chestnuts, hazelnuts, walnuts), onions, oranges, peas, poultry, prunes, raisins, salmon, sesame seeds, squash, sunflower seeds, sweet potatoes, tomatoes, tuna, watermelon, whole wheat

Vitamin B$_7$ (Biotin)

Biotin supports the myelin nerve sheath of the nervous system and can help calm anxiety and relieve insomnia. Biotin can be provided through the diet but is also produced by healthy intestinal flora. Antiseizure medications can lower biotin levels.

Sources: almonds, bananas, eggs, fish, green leafy vegetables, legumes, meat, mushrooms, nutritional yeast, raisins, soy, sweet potatoes, walnuts, whole grains

Vitamin B$_9$ (Folate/Folic Acid)

Folate is needed for the brain's energy production, helps make SAM-e (S-adenosyl-L-methionine), and is necessary for the production of dopamine and serotonin. Folic acid also helps in RNA and DNA production. Due to genetics, some people lack the ability to turn folic acid into its active form of L-5-methytetrahydrofolate (5-MTHF). Lack of 5-MTHF can interfere with neurotransmitters such as dopamine, serotonin, and norepinephrine. If you have persistent and worsening issues with anxiety, depression, and fatigue, ask your doctor about genetic testing.

Sources: almonds, artichokes, asparagus, avocados, barley, beans (especially garbanzos, lentils, soybeans), bee pollen, beets, blackberries, Brussels sprouts, cabbage, cantaloupe, chicken, dates, fenugreek seeds, fish (salmon, tuna), green leafy vegetables, lamb, nutritional yeast, nuts, oranges, papayas, pecans, plums, raisins, rice, rye, spinach, sunflower seeds, sweet potatoes, walnuts, whole wheat

Vitamin B$_{12}$ (Cobalamin)

Many people with neurological conditions are deficient in vitamin B$_{12}$. Most B$_{12}$ supplements are cyanocobalamin, which the body converts to methylcobalamin, but because not everyone is able to make this biological conversion, methylcobalamin is the preferred supplement. B$_{12}$ can help in the synthesis of RNA. A B$_{12}$ deficiency can manifest as fatigue and can progress to neuropathy if untreated.

Sources: alfalfa, bee pollen, dairy, eggs, ginseng, meat, nutritional yeast, sardines, sauerkraut, seaweeds, spirulina, sprouts, yogurt

Choline

Choline is a fatty acid necessary for the transmission of nerve impulses from the brain throughout the nervous system. It is not technically a vitamin, though it is usually grouped with the vitamin B complex. It regulates gallbladder function, liver function, and hormonal production and helps the breakdown of cholesterol, thus normalizing its levels. Choline is an essential part of the neurotransmitter acetylcholine and stimulates its production.

Sources: avocados, beans (especially garbanzos, lentils, peas, soybeans), beef, brown rice, cabbage, cauliflower, corn, cottage cheese, eggs, green beans, green leafy vegetables, lecithin, milk, peanuts, potatoes, whole grains

Lecithin

Lecithin is found in brain and nerve tissue and is the main dietary source of choline. It is a phospholipid that breaks down fat molecules so they are small enough to be carried in the blood to the cells, preventing arterial plaque. Both choline and lecithin have been found helpful in Parkinson's disease, dementia, and Alzheimers's. When buying lecithin, look for brands that contain at least 30 percent phosphatidylcholine.

Sources: avocados, beans, dairy, egg yolks, fish, nutritional yeast, soy, sunflower seeds, whole grains, yams, yogurt

Inositol

Inositol is not technically a vitamin but a sugar, though it is often grouped with the B-complex vitamins and is sometimes known as vitamin B_8. It helps reduce cholesterol, prevents hardening of the arteries, helps the liver metabolize fats, and has a calming effect. It aids internal cell communication and improves serotonin's effects. It is currently being used to treat ADHD, Alzheiner's, anxiety, autism, depression, bipolar disorder, obsessive-compulsive disorder, nerve pain, panic attacks, and schizophrenia.

Sources: avocados, beans, brown rice, cabbage, cantaloupe, eggs, fruits, green leafy vegetables, lecithin, liver, meat, nutritional yeast, nuts, oats, oranges, peanuts, raisins, seeds, soy, sprouts, whole grains

Vitamin C (Ascorbic Acid)

Vitamin C is an antioxidant that aids in the repair of the adrenal glands, among other tissues. It also aids in the production of interferon and antistress hormones, protects the body against the harmful effects of pollution, enhances immune system function, and improves the assimilation of iron.

Sources: acerola cherries, alfalfa sprouts, asparagus, avocado, bananas, bell peppers, blackberries, black currants, blueberries, Brazil nuts, broccoli, Brussels sprouts, cabbage, cantaloupe, cauliflower, chili peppers, collard greens, dandelion greens, gooseberries, grapefruit, green leafy vegetables, green peppers, guavas, hibiscus flowers, honeydew melons, kale, kidney beans, kiwis, kohlrabi, kumquats, lemons, limes, mangoes, oranges, papayas, parsley, pineapple, plums, radishes, raspberries, rose hips, sauerkraut, sorrel, spinach, strawberries, sweet potatoes, tomatoes, watercress, watermelon

Vitamin D

Vitamin D stimulates calcium absorption and supports bone growth and blood clotting. It improves nervous system function and, in particular, depression, as well as serotonin production. Since the body makes vitamin D through exposure to the sun, sunscreen can inhibit the production of vitamin D. Low levels of vitamin D can be a factor in depression and Alzheimer's.

Dietary sources of vitamin D are sparse; the following list of vegetables do provide small amounts of vitamin D.

Sources: alfalfa, basil, chickweed, bee pollen, eggs, fenugreek, green leafy vegetables, herring, horsetail, mullein, mushrooms, nettle, papaya, parsley, sardines, shiitakes, sunflower seeds and greens, sweet potatoes, watercress, wheatgrass

Vitamin E

Vitamin E is an antioxidant that improves circulation, aids tissue repair, promotes normal blood clotting, minimizes scarring, promotes fertility, and helps maintain healthy muscles, nerves, skin, and hair. It also inhibits the oxidation of lipids.

Sources: alfalfa, almonds, apples, asparagus, beans, beet greens, blackberries, blue-green algae, broccoli, cabbage, cherries, cold-pressed oils, dandelion greens, dulse, fish, green leafy vegetables (especially kale, lettuce, spinach, turnip greens, watercress), hazelnuts, kelp, leeks, nettle, nuts, oats, parsley, parsnips, peas, peanuts, pine nuts, purslane, quinoa, raspberry leaf, rose hips, seeds (chia, flax, hemp, pumpkin, sesame, sunflower), sprouted grains, squash, strawberries, sweet potatoes, tomatoes, walnuts, whole grains

Vitamin K

The "K" comes from "the Koagulation vitamin" (there already was a vitamin C), in tribute to this vitamin's role in aiding blood-clotting ability. Vitamin K also aids bone formation and helps convert glucose into glycogen for storage in the liver. Intestinal bacteria normally synthesize half of the vitamin K the body needs; the rest mustbe ingested.

Sources: alfalfa, broccoli, Brussels sprouts, cabbage, cauliflower, green leafy vegetables (especially dandelion greens and kale), kelp, nettles, oats, onions, rye, seaweed, shepherd's purse, soy, spinach, turnip greens, watercress, whole wheat

MINERALS

Boron

Boron helps the body metabolize calcium and magnesium and so is needed for strong bones. It also enhances brain function and mental alertness.

Sources: alfalfa, almonds, apples, beans, broccoli, cabbage, carrots, dates, grapes, green leafy vegetables, hazelnuts, kelp, peaches, pears, peas, prunes, raisins, soy, spinach, whole grains

Calcium

Calcium is key to the formation of bones, teeth, and muscles. It helps maintain a regular heartbeat, prevents muscle cramps, and enhances the transmission of nerve impulses. Calcium deficiency has linked to anxiety, depression, irritability, and insomnia. Most calcium supplements are made of chalk (calcium carbonate); a calcium chelate or citrate is more absorbable. The body requires vitamin D in order to assimilate calcium.

Sources: almonds, beans (especially black, garbanzo, pinto, soy, and white), beet greens, Brazil nuts, broccoli, carob powder, collards, dairy, dandelion greens, figs, fish (with bones: canned salmon, sardines, anchovies), green leafy vegetables (especially collards, kale, and mustard greens), hazelnuts, lentils, miso, molasses, oats, seaweeds (especially dulse, hiziki, kelp, kombu, and wakame), sesame seeds, sunflower seeds, tempeh, tofu, turnip greens, yogurt

Chromium

Chromium aids in metabolism of glucose, fats, and protein. It supports the function of insulin and helps stabilize blood sugar levels. In supplement form you would want to look for GTF chromium—glucose tolerance factor chromium—because it is the natural form of chromium and so more bioavailable.

Sources: apples, bananas, barley, basil, beans, beets, black pepper, broccoli, carrots, catnip, cloves, grapes, horsetail, kelp, licorice root, meat, mushrooms, nettles, nutritional yeast, nuts, oatstraw, oranges, raisins, red clover, rye, tomatoes, watercress, whole grains, yarrow

Germanium

Germanium improves immune system function and cellular oxygenation.

Sources: aloe vera, barley, broccoli, celery, chlorella, comfrey, eleuthero, garlic, ginseng, oats, shiitakes, suma, tomato

Iodine

Iodine is a trace mineral necessary for thyroid health and the prevention of goiter. It helps curb weight gain. Soy can inhibit iodine absorption.

Sources: asparagus, beans, bee pollen, beets, cabbage, carrots, fish, garlic, green leafy vegetables, onions, pineapple, sea salt, seaweed, sesame seeds, Swiss chard, turnip greens, whole wheat

Iron

Iron is essential in the blood to transport oxygen and for the production of hemoglobin. It also relieves fatigue. If iron levels are too low or high, pain, poor memory, and intolerance to cold can occur. Excessive iron can interfere with the heart muscle's contractions, cause free radical damage, and promote the oxidation of low-density lipoprotein (LDL) cholesterol.

Sources: almonds, apricots (dried), beans (especially black, garbanzo, lentils, lima, navy, pinto, soy, and split peas), blackberries, bran, burdock root, carrots, cherries, collards, green leafy vegetables (especially beet greens, kale, and spinach), green peppers, Jerusalem artichokes, liver, millet, miso, nettles, oats, onions, oysters, parsley, persimmons, prunes, pumpkin seeds, raisins, red meat, seaweed (especially dulse, hiziki, kelp, kombu, and nori), sesame seeds, shallots, squash, sunflower seeds, watercress, wheat bran, winter squash

Lithium

Lithium, a natural mineral, can help prevent depression (especially bipolar) and addiction and improve fertility. It also has antiviral properties.

Sources: cabbage, coriander, cumin, dulse, eggplant, green leafy vegetables, kelp, peppers, potatoes, tomatoes

Magnesium

Magnesium is necessary for bone structure and muscle and nerve function and helps convert the amino acid 5-HTP into serotonin. It also helps prevent and relax spasms. A deficiency in magnesium can contribute to many mental and emotional health issues, such as anxiety, ADHD, irritability, and bipolar conditions. It can also help with migraines, headaches, growing pains, fibromyalgia, restless leg, menstrual cramps, constipation, heart palpatations, muscle twitches, and some back and sciatic pain.

As a supplement, magnesium glycinate is very absorbable and less likely to be laxative than some other forms of magnesium. Magnesium gels and creams are also an option. Epsom salt baths are yet another method of assimilating magnesium.

Sources: alfalfa, almonds, apricots, artichokes, avocados, bananas, barley, beans (especially black-eyed peas, kidney beans, lentils, lima beans, soybeans, and split peas), Brazil nuts, broccoli, brown rice, buckwheat, cantaloupe, carrots, cashews, catnip, cauliflower, celery, chocolate (dark), cloves, corn, dates, fenugreek, figs, fish (fatty varieties), green leafy vegetables (especially beet greens, collards, dandelion, mustard greens, spinach, and Swiss chard), horsetail, mangoes, millet, mushrooms, nettles, oats, oranges, paprika, parsley, parsnips, peas, peaches, pecans, peppermint, peppers, pineapple, pine nuts, prunes, quinoa, raspberry leaf, red clover, rye, sage, seaweed (especially dulse, kelp, nori, and wakame), seeds (especially pumpkin, sesame, and sunflower), shepherd's purse, squash, strawberries, sweet potatoes, tofu, tomatoes, triticale, walnuts, watercress, watermelon, whole grains, wild rice, yarrow, yellow dock

Manganese

Manganese strengthens the tissue and linings of body structures (including bones) and improves memory, brain, and nerve function. It is needed for blood sugar balance and immune system function.

Sources: alfalfa, almonds, apples, apricots, avocados, bananas, beans, bee pollen, beets, blueberries, broccoli, brown rice, burdock root, carrots, catnip, celery, chamomile, chickweed, corn, dandelion greens, fennel seed, fenugreek, ginseng, green leafy vegetables, hops, lemongrass, mullein, nasturtium leaves, nuts, oats, parsley, peas, peppercorns, peppermint, persimmons, pineapple, pine nuts, prunes, raspberries (fruit and leaf), red clover, rose hips, rye, seaweed, seeds, shellfish, soy, sweet potatoes, walnuts, whole grains, yarrow, yellow dock

Methyl-Sulfonyl-Methane (MSM)

MSM is a form of organic sulfur. It helps prevent skin eruptions, thickens and beautifies hair, improves athletic recovery time, supports the elasticity of tissues, and enhances brain function.

Sources: aloe vera, asparagus, Brussels sprouts, eggs, garlic, kale, meat, onions, pine bark, pine needles, pine nuts

Molybdenum

Molybdenum is needed in tiny amounts for the metabolism of nitrogen. It promotes normal cell function and a healthy libido.

Sources: apricots, barley, beans (especially black eyed peas, lentils, lima beans, peas, and soybeans), beef liver, buckwheat, cantaloupe, carrots, dairy, eggs, garlic, green leafy vegetables, meat, raisins, strawberries, sunflower seeds, whole grains

Phosphorus

Phosphorus builds nerve strength, enhances mental capacity, and stimulates bone and hair growth. It helps generate cell energy and is a component of DNA. It is needed by all the organs of the body. It tends to be overabundant in Western diets.

Sources: almonds, asparagus, beans (especially garbanzos, peas, and soybeans), broccoli, buckwheat, corn, dairy, fish, garlic, green leafy vegetables (especially collards and kale), meat, nuts, parsnips, pumpkin seeds, sesame seeds, seaweeds (especially dulse), whole grains (especially wheat and rye)

Potassium

Potassium promotes tissue elasticity, supple muscles, regular heartbeat, and stable blood pressure. Cramps, muscle spasms, or a changeable personality can indicate a potassium deficiency.

Sources: almonds, apricots, avocados, bananas, beans, beets and their greens, blueberries, brown rice, buckwheat, cabbage, cantaloupe, carrots, catnip, currants, dates, dulse, figs, garlic, grapes, green leafy vegetables (especially spinach and Swiss chard), hops, horsetail, lentils, nettles, onions, oranges, papayas, peaches, plantains, pumpkin seeds, raisins, red clover, sage, seafood, skullcap, sunflower seeds, tomatoes, watermelon, winter squash

Selenium

Selenium inhibits the oxidation of fats. It protects the immune system by preventing free radicals and aiding in the production of antibodies. A selenium deficiency can manifest as negative moods, depression, or anxiety.

Sources: alfalfa, asparagus, barley, beets, black-eyed peas, Brazil nuts, broccoli, brown rice, burdock root, butter, cabbage, carrots, cashews, catnip, cayenne, celery, chamomile, chicken, chickweed, dairy products, dulse, eggs, fennel seed, fenugreek, fish (especially shellfish), garlic, ginseng, green leafy vegetables, hawthorn berries, honey, hops, horsetail, kelp, kombu, lemongrass, lentils, liver, milk thistle seeds, molasses, mushrooms, nettles, nutritional yeast, nuts, oatstraw, onions, parsley, peppermint, raspberry leaf, rose hips, seafood, seaweeds, soy, spinach, spirulina, squash, sunflower seeds, tomatoes, watercress, whole grains, yarrow, yellow dock

Silica

Silica is found in body structures such as myelin nerve sheathing, blood vessels, cartilage, ligaments, tendons, lungs, trachea, teeth, hair, and nails. It is insulating, helps warm the body, and promotes the electrical flow of energy via electrolytes. It improves elasticity and agility. A silicon deficiency can cause uncoordination, wrinkles, fungal infections, and erectile dysfunction.

Sources: alfalfa sprouts, almonds, apples, apricots, asparagus, barley, beer, beets, brown rice, burdock root, carrots, cauliflower, celery, cherries, cucumbers, figs, flaxseed, grapes, green beans, green leafy vegetables (especially dandelion greens, lettuce, nettles, spinach, and Swiss chard), hempseed, horseradish, horsetail, Jerusalem artichoke, kelp, leeks, oats, parsnips, peppers, pumpkins, radishes, red lentils, sprouts, strawberries, sunflower seeds, tomatoes, watermelon, wild rice

Sodium

Sodium purifies and cools the blood and supports the formation of saliva, bile, and pancreatic fluids.

Sources: apples, apricots, asparagus, beets, celery, coconuts, garbanzo beans, goat's milk, green leafy vegetables (especially beet greens, dandelion greens, spinach, Swiss chard, and watercress), millet, okra, olives, prunes, raisins, seaweeds, sesame seeds, strawberries, sweet potatoes, tomatoes, turnips

Sulfur

Sulfur aids in the digestion of fats and helps prevent blood platelet aggregation. It imparts a glow to the skin. It improves skin elasticity, supports tissue repair, prevents scarring, reduces lactic acid buildup, and improves athletic recovery time. It also aids liver detoxification. Some sulfur-rich foods can be gas forming; eating them with sodium-rich foods can relieve this.

Sources: apples, apricots, arugula, asparagus, beans, blue-green algae, broccoli, Brussels sprouts, cabbage, carrots, cauliflower, cayenne, celery, durian, eggs, garlic, green leafy vegetables (especially kale, mustard greens, nasturtium leaves, Swiss chard, and watercress), hempseed, horseradish, nuts, onions, peaches, prunes, pumpkin seeds, radishes, soy, spirulina, turnips, whole grains

Vanadium

Vanadium is needed for the formation of teeth and bones. It aids growth, reproduction, and cellular metabolism. It plays a role in controlling blood sugar levels and prevents the development of high LDL cholesterol.

Sources: buckwheat, dill, oats, olives, parsley, radishes, shellfish, soy, string beans, whole grains

Zinc

Zinc is needed for adrenal strength, strong immunity, sexuality, and fertility. It also improves the senses of taste and smell. Adequate zinc is necessary to prevent or remedy acne, hair loss, skin disorders, low sperm count, poor wound healing, and poor eyesight.

Sources: adzuki beans, alfalfa, almonds, beans, bee pollen, black pepper, Brazil nuts, brown rice, buckwheat, burdock root, cashews, cayenne, chamomile, chickweed, chocolate (dark),coconuts, corn, dandelion greens, dill seed, fennel seed, garlic, hops, kelp, macadamia nuts, meat, milk thistle seeds, mushrooms, nettles, nutritional yeast, oats, onions, oysters, parsley, peanuts, peas, pecans, peppermint, pine nuts, poppyseeds, pumpkin seeds, rose hips, rye, sage, sarsaparilla, sesame seeds, shellfish, soy, spinach, spirulina, sunflower seeds, walnuts, whole grains

ESSENTIAL FATTY ACIDS (EFAS)

EFAs improve skin and hair, lower blood pressure and cholesterol levels, and reduce the risk of blood clots. They are found in high concentrations in the brain, and all cells, including those involved in the production of hormones, need them.

Sources: evening primrose oil, flaxseed, purslane, sesame seeds, sunflower seeds

Omega-3 Fatty Acids

Omega-3 fatty acids are found in cell membranes and are necessary for the production of anti-inflammatory prostaglandins, but they cannot be synthesized in the body, so we must take them in through our diet. Perhaps the two best-known omega-3s are docosahexaenoic acid (DHA) and eicosapentaenoic acid (EPA); bipolar disorder, depression, and ADHD can signal a deficiency of these omega-3s. Omega-3s can reduce inflammation in the body, including the brain. DHA is needed to build the membrane that surrounds the brain, including the synapses. This nutrient is essential in promoting positive moods for new mothers who may be inclined to postpartum depression. EPA can reduce pain and swelling and help alleviate depression.

Note: It's best to avoid omega-3 supplementation for seven to ten days before surgery, as it can have blood-thinning properties.

Sources: beans, black currant seed oil, blue-green algae, borage seed oil, cabbage, evening primrose oil, fish (oily varieties like mackerel and salmon), green leafy vegetables, hazelnuts, pecans, pine nuts, purslane, seeds (chia, flax, hemp, pumpkin, and sesame), soy, spinach, squash, walnuts, wheat

Omega-6 Fatty Acids

Like omega-3 fatty acids, omega-6 fatty acids cannot be synthesized in the body. A deficiency of omega-6 fatty acids can contribute to eczema, hair loss, liver degeneration, suseptability to infections, infertility in men, and miscarriage in women.

Sources: beans, black currant seed oil, borage seed oil, corn, evening primrose oil, fish (especially herring, salmon, sardines, salmon, oysters, trout, and tuna), pumpkin seeds, sesame seeds, vegetable oils, whole grains

Gamma-Linolenic Acid (GLA)

GLA helps lower cholesterol and blood pressure. It inhibits the formation of blood clots, improves mood, and can aid in weight loss.

Sources: black currant seed oil, borage seed oil, chia seed, flaxseed, hempseed, perilla seed, soy, walnuts

AMINO ACIDS

Amino acids are organic compounds that represent the final stage of protein hydrolysis. Ten amino acids are considered essential, meaning they must be acquired through the diet, because the body does not manufacture adequate amounts of them.

The Essential Amino Acids

Arginine	Methionine
Histidine	Phenylalanine
Isoleucine	Threonine
Leucine	Tryptophan
Lysine	Valine

Arginine

Arginine enhances immune function, improves liver function, is a component of seminal fluid, and accelerates the repair of tissue. It is also necessary for muscle building.

Sources: apples, apricots, beans, berries, coconuts, dairy, eggplant, fish, meat, nuts, pineapple, seeds, strawberries, tomatoes, vegetables (all except celery and turnips), whole grains

Carnitine

Carnitine is not considered a true amino acid but has a similar chemical structure. It transports fats that are burned as energy, helping to minimize fat buildup in the liver and heart. It helps reduce fatigue, increases HDLs, reduces blood ketone levels, and may improve the motility and fertility of sperm. It may improve liver function in cases of alcohol abuse. Some forms of kidney disease may benefit from carnitine. One way to increase carnitine levels is to increase consumption of lysine-rich foods. It has not yet been discovered in a vegetable source. As a supplement, it is best taken in capsules on an empty stomach; only the L-form should be used.

Sources: dairy, fish, meat

Cysteine

Cysteine improves skin texture and is needed for B vitamin utilization. It is considered an antioxidant, helping to protect the body from the ravages of pollution.

Sources: beans, Brazil nuts, eggs, meat, soy, whole wheat, yogurt

Glutamic Acid

Glutamic acid is a neurotransmitter that increases the firing of neurons. It helps in the metabolism of fats and sugars and helps potassium cross the blood-brain barrier.

Sources: dairy, dates, eggs, fish, meats, shiitakes

Glutamine

Glutamine is an amino acid that aids in the production of GABA and elevates glutathione levels. It strengthens immune health, hastens recovery time, and rejuvenates muscles weakened by illness and stress. It also helps balance acid/alkaline levels, is needed for the production of RNA and DNA, and promotes mental alertness, focus, and concentration.

Sources: beans, cabbage, dairy, eggs, fish, green leafy vegetables, nuts, oats, parsley, seaweed, seeds, soy, spinach

Glutathione

Glutathione, an antioxidant that aids liver cleansing, is composed of three amino acids: cysteine, glutamic acid, and glycine. Glutathione is not technically an amino acid but is considered a tripeptide. It transforms harmful peroxides, including hydrogen and lipid peroxides, into harmless molecules. It has been found to have antiaging properties and helps with carbohydrate metabolism. It is not well absorbed orally, so a liposomal source that is fat soluble would be more absorbable.

Sources: almonds, asparagus, avocados, baru nuts, broccoli, cantaloupe, carrots, garlic, milk thistle seed, okra, onions, peaches, potatoes, spinach, sprouted seeds, strawberries, tomatoes, turmeric, walnuts, watermelon, winter squash

Glycine

Glycine is needed for the synthesis of bile acids and nucleic acids and is used in the formation of RNA and DNA. High levels are found in the connective tissues and skin. It is an important component of the antioxidant glutathione, and when combined with ornithine and arginine, it may promote healing.

Sources: asparagus, avocados, beans, bone broth, cabbage, dairy, meat, oats, seafood, seaweed, watercress, wheat germ

Histidine

Histidine is a metal-chelating agent. It transports nutrients and is needed to produce red and white blood cells.

Sources: apples, beans, dairy, fish, meat, nuts, papayas, pineapple, seeds, vegetables (all except celery, radishes, and turnips)

Isoleucine

Isoleucine helps make biochemical components that produce energy. It is needed for the production of hemoglobin and helps regulate blood sugar levels.

Sources: almonds, apples, apricots, beans, cashews, dairy, dates, figs, fish, lentils, meat, nuts, peaches, pears, persimmons, rye, seeds, strawberries, tofu, tomatoes, vegetables (all except celery, lettuce, and radishes)

Leucine

Leucine stimulates protein synthesis in muscles, aids in healing wounds of the bones and skin, and is necessary for growth.

Sources: apples, apricots, dairy, dates, figs, legumes, meat, nuts, peaches, pears, seeds, strawberries, tomatoes, vegetables (all except celery, lettuce, and radishes), whole grains

Lysine

Lysine supports the absorption of calcium from the intestinal tract and helps in the production of antibodies, enzymes, hormones, collagen, and bones. It inhibits the replication of sores caused by the herpes virus.

Sources: aloe, apples, apricots, avocados, bananas, beans, cantaloupe, dates, eggs, figs, grapefruit, meat, nuts, oranges, papayas, peaches, pears, persimmons, pineapple, quinoa, seeds (especially pumpkin), soy, strawberries, tomatoes, vegetables (all), whole grains, yogurt

Methionine

Methionine is an antioxidant that aids digestion, protects against radiation, minimizes fat buildup in liver, and reduces histamine reaction.

Sources: apples, apricots, avocados, bananas, Brazil nuts, cantaloupe, dates, eggs, figs, garlic, lentils, nuts, oranges, papayas, peaches, pears, persimmons, pineapple, rice, sesame seeds, soy, strawberries, sunflower seeds, vegetables (all), whole grains, yogurt

Ornithine

Ornithine aids the release of growth hormones, thus helping the metabolism of fat. It is needed for immune and liver function and promotes the healing of tissues. It scavenges free radicals.

Sources: dairy products, eggs, fish, meat

Phenylalanine

Phenylalanine helps in the formation of neurotransmitters, including norepinephrine and dopamine, and is a precursor to tyrosine. It can help relieve pain and depression.

Sources: almonds, apples, apricots, avocados, bananas, beans (especially garbanzos, lentils, lima beans, and soybeans), beets, carrots, dairy, figs, fish, meat, nuts, parsley, peaches, pears, persimmons, pineapple, seeds, strawberries, tomatoes, vegetables (especially lettuce and radishes), whole grains

Serine

Serine helps in the metabolism of fats and supports muscle growth and a healthy immune system. The D form of serine protects nerve cells of the brain.

Sources: dairy products, eggs, meat

Taurine

Taurine is a component of all the other amino acids and aids in bile production. Though it is not found in vegetable protein, the body will synthesize taurine as long as adequate vitamin B_6 is present.

Sources: beef, eggs, poultry, seaweed, shellfish, tuna

Theanine

Theanine is an amino acid that helps protect the brain from being overstimulated. It improves cognition and memory and promotes both alertness during the day and deep sleep at night. It also can help calm heart rate during times of acute stress.

Source: green tea

Threonine

Threonine supports the health of tooth enamel, elastin, and collagen. It minimizes fat in liver and stimulates the immune system.

Sources: apples, apricots, beans, cottage cheese, dates, figs, nuts, peaches, pears, persimmons, seeds, strawberries, vegetables (all except celery and lettuce), wheat germ, whole grains

Tryptophan and 5 HTP

Tryptophan is needed for niacin, melatonin, and serotonin production. It can encourage healthy sleep, improve memory, and elevate moods. Those with bipolar conditions often respond well to tryptophan supplementation; it can improve the response to lithium supplementation.

Tryptophan is converted into 5 HTP, which then becomes serotonin. Both help decrease fibromyalgia, pain, and depression. They have been found to affect the prefrontal cortex, which is the part of the brain associated with positive mood, restraint, and impulsiveness.

As a supplement, tryptophan helps those who have trouble staying asleep. A tryptophan supplement is best taken with a carbohydrate snack. Supplementation of 5-HTP can help decrease anxiety and panic. They should not be taken along with SSRI (serotonin reuptake inhibiting drugs) or MAOI drugs (like Prozac), unless under medical supervision.

Sources of Tryptophan: alfalfa, almonds, avocados, bananas, beans (especially adzuki, mung, and soy), brown rice, cashews, cheddar cheese, chicken, cottage cheese, dark chocolate, dates, durian, egg whites, figs, fish, grapefruit, milk, nuts, oats, oranges, papayas, peaches, pears, persimmons, pineapple, seeds (especially pumpkin and sunflower), strawberries, tuna, turkey, green leafy vegetables (all), whole grains

Sources of 5 HTTP: chanterelle mushrooms, couch grass, Griffonia simplicifolia seeds, quack grass, and Saint John's wort.

Tyramine

Tyramine helps regulate blood pressure. Blocking this compound can help relieve depression. Excessive tyramine can contribute to migraine headaches.

Note: Avoid taking tyramine as a supplement if you are using MAOIs.

Sources: aged cheeses, apple cider vinegar, avocados, bananas, beer, dates, deli meats (bologna and salami), eggplant, fermented foods, kimchi, processed meats, lemons, miso, nuts, organ meats, pickled vegetables, pineapple, plums, sauerkraut, smoked foods, tangerines, tofu, tomatoes

Tyrosine

Tyrosine is a precursor to the neurotransmitters norepinephrine and dopamine, which help mood regulation, and is needed for proper adrenal, thyroid, and nervous system function. It is especially helpful for controlling depression and anxiety and improving mood.

Sources: alfalfa, almonds, apples, apricots, asparagus, avocados, bananas, beans, beets, bell peppers, carrots, cherries, chicken, cucumbers, dairy products, eggs, figs, fish, leeks, lettuce, lima beans, meat, parsley, pumpkin seeds, sesame seeds, soy, spinach, spirulina, strawberries, sunflower seeds, turkey, watercress, watermelon, wheat germ, yogurt

Valine

Valine is stimulating and can help curb addictions. It also helps build muscles and aids in tissue repair.

Sources: apples, apricots, cheese, dates, figs, fish, legumes, meats, mushrooms, nuts, peaches, pears, persimmons, seeds, soy, strawberries, vegetables (all except celery and lettuce), whole grains

FLAVONOIDS

Flavonoids are a group of more than five thousand powerful antioxidants. Bioflavonoids—that is, the flavonoids that are biologically active—enhance the assimilation of vitamin C, thereby helping to protect the structure of the capillaries, cell membranes, and blood vessels. They have an antibacterial effect, improve circulation, lower cholesterol, and stimulate bile production.

Sources: apples, apricots, bell pepper, berries (all), black currants, buckwheat, cacao, cantaloupe, cherries, citrus fruit and skins (inner rind), grapefruit, grapes (red, with seeds), kale, lemon balm, onions, onions (red), papayas, parsley, peppers, persimmons, pine bark, plums, pomegranates, prunes, rose hips, soy, tomatoes, walnuts, wine (red)

Quercetin

Quercetin is an antioxidant with anti-inflammatory and antiviral properties.

Sources: apples, blue-green algae, broccoli, buckwheat, cherries, cilantro, citrus fruit peels, clover blossoms, dill weed, eucalyptus leaves, fennel leaves, garlic, grapes (red, with skin), green leafy vegetables, lovage, onions, pansies, ragweed pollen, rinds and barks from wild fruits, watercress, wine (red)

Rutin

Rutin enhances the elasticity of veins and the assimilation of vitamin C.

Sources: apricots, blackberries, buckwheat, cherries, citrus peels (the inner white portion), ginkgo, hawthorn berries, rose hips, yarrow

Proanthocyanidins and Anthocyanosides

These flavonoids include cyanidin, delphinidin, malvidin, and petunidin. They strengthen capillaries and collagen and prevent inflammation, diminish allergy symptoms, and help prevent varicosities.

Sources: bilberries, blueberries, citrus fruit seeds, ginkgo, grape seeds, pine bark

Hesperidin

Hesperidin helps lower LDL cholesterol and elevate HDL cholesterol. It also has anti-inflammatory effects.

Sources: berries, grapefruit, lemon, oranges

Catechin

Catechin inhibits viral infection. It is antioxidant and helps protect against lipid peroxidation, thus suppressing the growth of many types of cancers.

Sources: berries, cacao, dark grapes, red wine.

PROBIOTICS

Probiotics are the healthful, "friendly" bacteria that normally reside in our gut. They help us digest our food and aid in the formation of vitamin K, biotin, and other essential nutrients, as well as supporting the production of neurotransmitters and hormones. Research has shown that gut and brain health are intimately connected.

Poor diet, stress, and especially antibiotics can decimate our intestinal flora. Eating probiotic foods and/or taking probiotic supplements can help in its restoration and improve conditions such as depression, anxiety, autism, and Alzheimer's.

Source: fermented foods (buttermilk, kefir, kimchi, miso, sauerkraut, yogurt, and so on)

OTHER IMPORTANT NUTRIENTS

Alpha-Lipoic Acid

This antioxidant improves the utilization of glucose, lowers cholesterol, and reduces the oxidation of LDL cholesterol. It may be neuroprotective.

Sources: beets, broccoli, Brussels sprouts, organ meats, potatoes, spinach, tomatoes

Allyl Sulfides

Allyl sulfides stimulate glutathione levels and S-transferase, an enzyme of detoxification.

Sources: chives, garlic, leeks, onions

Coenzyme Q10

Coenzyme Q10 (also known as ubiquinone) is an antioxidant that strengthens the heart muscle, lowers blood pressure, reduces the effects of aging, and relaxes constricted blood vessels. It also appears to protect neurons from neurotoxic agents.

Sources: almonds, broccoli, fish (oily), meat, salmon, sardines, spinach, whole grains, yogurt

Fructo-Oligosaccharides

Fructo-oligosaccharides are chains of sugar molecules that enhance beneficial bacteria in the intestines. They also decrease putrefactive substances, support healthy intestinal flora, promote bowel regularity, improve immune function, and support liver function.

Sources: artichokes, asparagus, bananas, barley, chicory root, garlic, Jerusalem artichoke, onions, tomatoes, yacon

Phosphatidylserine

Phosphatidylserine is the most abundant phospholipid in the brain, though it tends to decline as we age. It helps maintain the integrity of brain tissue and the fluidity of cellular membranes, thus benefiting neuron transmission. It also boosts norepinephrine, dopamine, and serotonin levels.

It is manufactured by the body, but requires diet for supplementation.

Sources: beef liver, chicken, eggs, soy (especially soy lecithin), white beans

Resveratrol

Resveratrol is a polyphenol antioxidant with anticancer properties.

Sources: grape skins, Japanese knotweed, peanuts, pine nuts

Ribonucleic Acid (RNA)

RNA is associated with the control of cellular chemical activities. In layman's terms, it carries information, signals, and messages through the body.

Sources: asparagus, beef, beets, green leafy vegetables, lentils, mushrooms, nuts, radishes, seafood

Gamma Aminobutyric Acid (GABA)

GABA is an important neurotransmitter that aids relaxation and promotes better mood and sleep. It helps us feel calm, peaceful, and less affected by feeling overwhelmed. As a supplement, it works best when taken with vitamin B_6.

Sources: broccoli, cabbage, fava beans, green tea, nuts, spinach

N-Acetylcysteine (NAC)

Derived from the amino acid cysteine, this high sulfur compound stimulates production of glutathione. It has strong anti-inflammatory properties. NAC helps detoxify the body of environmental pollutants, including heavy metals.

Sources: beans, beef, broccoli, eggs, fish, onions, sunflower seeds, yogurt

Resources

In this chapter you will find information about organizations that offer support for various aspects of mental and emotional health. You will also find reliable resources for purchasing and gaining a broader understanding of many of the natural remedies suggested in this book.

Herb Education Resources

American Botanical Council
www.herbalgram.org
Publishes Herbalgram *and sells herbal books.*

American Herbalists Guild
www.americanherbalistsguild.com/
Offers a member directory of peer-reviewed herbal practitioners.

American Herb Association
www.ahaherb.com
Provides listing of herb schools throughout the country and an excellent newsletter.

Erowid
www.erowid.com
Research and education on the safety and pitfalls of psychedelics and other drug research.

Herbal Healing with Brigitte Mars

https://sevenroots.com/herbal-healing-with-brigitte-mars/

An online course about herbalism offered through Seven Roots.

United Plant Savers

www.unitedplantsavers.org

Group that promotes awareness about rare and endangered species and offers a great newsletter.

Mental Health Resources

National Institute of Mental Health

www.nimh.nih.gov

This is the lead federal agency for research on mental disorders.

World Federation for Mental Health

https://wfmh.global/

International organization founded to advance, among all peoples and nations, the prevention of mental and emotional disorders, the proper treatment and care of those with such disorders, and the promotion of mental health.

Resources for Buying Herbs and Supplies

Allergy Research Group

www.allergyresearchgroup.com

Sells homeopathic products for specific allergens, as well as a wide variety of supplements and herbs.

Asia Natural Products

www.drkangformulas.com

Sells quality Asian herbs.

Bach Original Flower Remedies

www.bachremedies.com

Distributors of Rescue Remedy and other Bach flower essences.

Boiron Homeopathics

www.boironusa.com

Offers a complete line of homeopathic products.

Frontier Natural Products Co-Op

www.frontiercoop.com

Offers herbs and herbal products.

Herb Pharm

www.herb-pharm.com

Makers of excellent-quality herbal tinctures.

Strictly Medicinal Seeds

https://strictlymedicinalseeds.com

Offers an excellent selection of medicinal herb seeds and seedlings.

Mountain Rose Herbs

www.mountainroseherbs.com

Sells herbs and herbal products such as strainers, empty tea bags, and tincture bottles.

Planetary Herbals

www.planetaryherbals.com

Sells herbal remedies based on the work of Michael Tierra, C.A., N.D.

StarWest Botanicals

www.starwest-botanicals.com

Offers herbs and herbal products.

Bibliography

Ameet, Aggarwal. *Heal Your Body, Cure Your Mind: Leaky Gut, Adrenal Fatigue, Liver Detox, Mental Health, Anxiety, Depression, Disease & Trauma: Mindfulness, Holistic Therapies, Diet, Nutrition & Food*. Africa: Foundation for Integrated Medicine in Africa, 2017.

Anderson, Nina, and Howard Peiper. *A.D.D.: The Natural Approach: Help for Children with Attention Deficit Disorder and Hyperactivity*. Sheffield, Mass.: Safe Goods Publishing, 2004.

Arbett, Lorenzo. *Kicking the Depression Habit*. New York: Prema Publishing, 1988.

Ayan, Jordan. *Aha! 10 Ways to Free Your Creative Spirit and Find Your Great Ideas*. New York: Random House, 1997.

Barrett, Susan. *It's All in Your Head: A Guide to Understanding Your Brain and Boosting Your Brain Power*. Minneapolis: Free Spirit Publishing, 1985.

Black, Dean. *Four Steps to an Alert and Active Mind*. Springville, Utah: Tapestry Press, 1989.

Bloomfield, Harold H. *Healing Anxiety with Herbs: Featuring a Natural Self-Healing Program to Relieve Stress, Promote Sleep & Maximize Performance*. New York: HarperCollins, 1998.

Bragg, Paul, and Patricia Bragg. *Build Powerful Nerve Force: It Controls Your Life—Keep It Healthy*. Santa Barbara, Calif.: Health Science, 2007.

Brown, Richard P., Patricia L. Gerbarg, and Philip R. Muskin. *How to Use Herbs, Nutrients and Yoga in Mental Health Care*. New York: W. W. Norton and Company, 2009.

Butler, Gillian, and Tony Hope. *Managing Your Mind: The Mental Fitness Guide*. New York: Oxford University Press, 1995.

Challem, Jack. *The Food-Mood Solution: All-Natural Ways to Banish Anxiety, Depression, Anger, Stress, Overeating and Alcohol and Drug Problems—and Feel Good Again*. Hoboken, N.J.: John Wiley and Sons, 2007.

Colodzin, Benjamin. *How to Survive Trauma: A Program for War Veterans and Survivors of Rape, Assault, Abuse and Environmental Disasters*. Barrytown, N.Y.: Stanton Hill Press, 1993.

Cousens, Gabriel, and Mark Mayell. *Depression-Free for Life: An All-Natural 5-Step Plan to Reclaim Your Zest for Living*. New York: Harper-Collins, 2000.

DeFelice, Karen. *Enzymes for Autism and Other Neurological Conditions*. Minneapolis: Thundersnow Interactive Publications, 2003.

Emery, Gary, and James Campbell. *Rapid Relief from Emotional Distress: A New Clinically Proven Method for Getting Over Depression and Other Emotional Problems without Prolonged or Expensive Therapy*. New York: Rawson Associates, 1986.

Gawain, Shakti. *Creative Visualization: Use the Power of Your Imagination to Create What You Want in Your Life*. Novato, Calif.: New World Library, 2002.

Germano, Carl, and William Cabot. *Nature's Pain Killers: Nutritional and Alternative Therapies for Chronic Pain Relief*. New York: Kensington Publishing, 2000.

Gladstar, Rosemary. *Herbs for Reducing Stress and Anxiety*. Pownal, Vt.: Storey Books, 1999.

Hickland, Catherine. *The 30-Day Heartbreak Cure: Getting Over Him and Back Out There One Month from Today*. New York: Simon and Schuster, 2009.

Hoffer, Abram, and Morton Walker. *Smart Nutrients: A Guide to Nutrients That Can Prevent and Reverse Senility*. Garden City Park, N.Y.: Avery Publishing, 1994.

Hoffmann, David. *Successful Stress Control: The Natural Way*. Rochester, Vt.: Thorsons Publishers, 1987.

Hunt, Douglas. *No More Fears: From Crippling Phobias to the Jitters, Fight Your Fears with Nutrition!* New York: Warner Books, 1988.

Ingram, Cass. *The Cannabis Cure: Perfect Wellness through the Powers of Whole Food Raw Cannabis*. Vernon Hills, Ill.: Knowledge House Publishers, 2016.

Katz, Lawrence C., and Manning Rubin. *Keep Your Brain Alive: 83 Neurobic Exercises to Help Prevent Memory Loss and Increase Mental Fitness*. New York: Workman Publishing, 1999.

Kemper, Kathi, J. *Mental Health, Naturally: The Family Guide to a Holistic Care for a Healthy Mind and Body*. Elk Grove Village, Ill.: American Academy of Pediatrics, 2010.

Kiew Kit, Wong. *The Complete Book of Chinese Medicine: A Holistic Approach to Physical, Emotional and Mental Health*. Kedah, Malaysia: Cosmos Internet Publishing, 2002.

Kircher, Tamara. *Herbs for the Soul: Emotional Healing with Chinese and Western Herb and Bach Flower Remedies*. London: Hammersmith, 2001.

Kirsta, Alix. *The Book of Stress Survival: Identifying and Reducing the Stress in Your Life*. New York: Simon and Schuster, 1986.

Kurn, Sidney J. *Herbs and Nutrients for Neurological Disorders: Treatment Strategies for Alzheimer's, Parkinson's, Stroke, Multiple Sclerosis, Migraines, Seizures*. Rochester, Vt.: Healing Arts Press, 2016.

Larre, Claude, and Elisabeth Rochat de la Vallée. *The Seven Emotions: Psychology and Health in Ancient China*. Cambridge, England: Monkey Press, 1996.

Larson, Joan Mathews. *7 Weeks to Emotional Healing: Proven Natural Formulas for Eliminating Depression, Anxiety, Fatigue, and Anger from Your Life*. New York: Ballantine Publishing Group, 1999.

Levine, Peter A. *Waking the Tiger: Healing Trauma*. Berkeley, Calif.: North Atlantic Books, 1997.

Levine, Peter G. *Stronger after Stroke: Your Roadmap to Recovery*. New York: Demos Health, 2018.

Mayell, Mark. *Natural Energy: A Consumer's Guide to Legal, Mind-Altering, and Mood-Brightening Herbs and Supplements*. New York: Three Rivers Press, 1998.

Medina, John. *Depression: How It Happens, How It's Healed*. Hong Kong: New Harbinger Publications, Inc., 1998.

Murray, Michael T. *Natural Alternatives to Prozac*. New York: William Morrow and Company, 1996.

O'Bannon, Kathleen, C.N.C. *The Anger Cure: A Step-by-Step Program to Reduce Anger, Rage, Negativity, Violence and Depression in Your Life*. Laguna Beach, Calif.: Basic Health Publications, 2007.

Permutter, David, and Austin Perlmutter. *Brain Wash: Detox Your Mind for Clearer Thinking, Deeper Relationships, and Lasting Happiness*. New York: Little, Brown, Spark, 2020.

Procyk, Anne. *Nutritional Treatments to Improve Mental Health Disorders: Non-Pharmaceutical Interventions for Depression, Anxiety, Bipolar & ADHD.* Eau Claire, Wisc.: PESI Publishing, 2018.

Russo, Etan. *Handbook of Psychotropic Herbs: A Scientific Analysis of Herbal Remedies for Psychiatric Conditions.* Binghamton, N.Y.: Haworth Press, 2001.

Sachs, Judith. *Nature's Prozac: Natural Therapies and Techniques to Rid Yourself of Anxiety, Depression, Panic Attacks and Stress.* Englewood Cliffs, N.J.: Prentice Hall, 1997.

Schnyer, Rosa, and Bob Flaws. *Chinese Medicine Cures Depression.* Berkshire, England: Foulsham Publishing, 2000.

Simontacchi, Carol. *The Crazy Makers: How the Food Industry Is Destroying Our Brains and Harming Our Children.* New York: Jeremy Tharcher/Penguin, 2007.

Stone, Thomas A. *Cure by Crying: How to Cure Your Own Depression, Nervousness, Headaches, Violent Temper, Insomnia, Marital Problems, Addictions by Uncovering Your Repressed Memories.* Des Moines: Cure by Crying, Inc., 1995.

Teitelbaum, Jacob. *Pain Free 1-2-3: A Proven Program for Eliminating Chronic Pain Now.* New York: McGraw-Hill, 2005.

Tolle, Eckhart. *The Power of Now: A Guide to Spiritual Enlightenment.* Novato, Calif.: New World Library, 1999.

Walker, Peter. *Complex-PTSD: From Surviving to Thriving.* Contra Costa, Calif.: Azure Coyote Publishing, 2013.

Wills-Brandon, Carla. *Natural Mental Health: How to Take Control of Your Own Emotional Well-Being.* Carlsbad, Calif.: Hay House, 2000.

Acknowledgments

From Brigitte

There are many to thank for the birthing of this book. I would like to express my gratitude to my coauthor, Chrystle Fiedler; to our agent, Marilyn Allen from the Allen Literary Agency; and to Inner Traditions, especially to my editors Meghan MacLean and Nancy Ringer, cover artist Aaron Davis, Jon Graham, and the entire production, sales, and marketing team. I am also grateful to Rosemary Gladstar for the beautiful foreword. Loving thanks to Bethy Love Light, my mom, Rita Smookler, Matthew Becker, Marjy Berkman, Mindy Green, Feather Jones, Valerie Blackenship, Lilja Oddsdottir, Lila Simoncini, Amelia Passer, Laura Lamun, Charles Roberts, Briggs Wallis, and Roy Upton. Blessings and thanks to Martina Hoffmann, Kimba Arem, Donnie Curren, Justin Bilancieri, Rachael Carlevale, Dr. Rob Ivker, Ed Bauman, Christine Martinez, Naropa University, Miss Hall's School, The Urantia Foundation, Tonics, and KGNU radio. And thanks to the dearly departed: William LeSassier, Rosemary Woodruff Leary, Terence McKenna, Roberto Venosa, Red Elk, and Morton Smookler.

From Chrystle

Much appreciation and thanks to Brigitte Mars, the best coauthor a writer could ever ask for; to my superstar agent, Marilyn Allen of the Allen Literary Agency; and to Rosemary Gladstar for her wonderful foreword. Many thanks to everyone at Inner Traditions, especially editor Meghan MacLean, copy editor Nancy Ringer, cover artist Aaron Davis, and the entire production, sales, and marketing team.

Wishing you all so many blessings!

Index

About the Authors

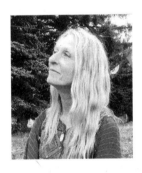

Brigitte Mars, A.H.G.

Brigitte Mars, A.H.G., has been an herbalist and natural health consultant for more than fifty years. She teaches herbal medicine at Naropa University. She has also taught in Iceland, Germany, England, Costa Rica, Colombia, and Mexico; at institutions such as the Omega Institute, Esalen, Kripalu, Sivananda Yoga Ashram, and the Mayo Clinic; and at the Unify, Arise, Envision, Burning Man, Tribal Visions, and Sister Winds festivals. She is a professional member of the American Herbalists Guild and is known by many as an eternal flower.

Brigitte is the author of many books, including *Addiction-Free Naturally, The Sexual Herbal, The Desktop Guide to Herbal Medicine, Natural First Aid, Healing Herbal Teas, Rawsome!,* and *Beauty by Nature,* and she is the coauthor of *The Country Almanac of Home Remedies* and *The HempNut Cookbook.* Her latest projects are a phone app called iPlant and an online course on herbal medicine.

To learn more about Brigitte's work, visit
brigittemars.com.

Chrystle Fiedler

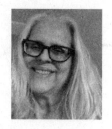

Chrystle Fiedler is the coauthor with Brigitte Mars of *The Country Almanac of Home Remedies*. She is also the author of *The Complete Idiot's Guide to Natural Remedies* and the coauthor of *Beat Sugar Addiction Now!, Beat Sugar Addiction Now! Cookbook,* and *The Complete Guide to Beating Sugar Addiction.* Chrystle also writes the Natural Remedies Mystery series for Gallery Books/Simon & Schuster, including the titles *Death Drops, Scent to Kill, Garden of Death,* and *Dandelion Dead.*

Chrystle's articles featuring health, wellness, and natural remedies have appeared in many national publications, including *USA Today, Woman's Day, Prevention, Mother Earth Living, Natural Health, Spirituality & Health, Vegetarian Times, AARP: The Magazine, Better Homes & Gardens,* and *Remedy.*

Chrystle is passionate about nature, animal welfare advocacy, and traveling.

To learn more about Chrystle's work, visit **chrystlefiedlerbooks.com.**